The Secrets to Intermittent Fasting: How You Can Stay Healthy, Slow Down the Aging Process, and Have a Lot of Energy

I0429592

By Malik Johnson

Table of Contents

Chapter 1: An Introduction To Intermittent Fasting:

Are you like millions of people out there who've tried numerous diets and wellness plans, from low-calorie, to low-fat and high-carb, from extreme calorie restriction, to eating 6 frequent meals, and found that despite all of the promises and the supposed "evidence", each one was just as ineffective as the last?

Like many people, you're probably sick of all the hype. The last thing you want to put your time and energy into is yet another diet! If so, that's great, because what I'm about to share with you is not a diet. It's not some brand new invention of the fitness world and it's not another new health fad based on crazy, unfounded claims. Instead, it's a secret to weight loss, health, youth, vitality, and longevity that is rooted in ancient knowledge of the way our bodies heal, repair, and rejuvenate themselves.

This secret was known and used by the great figures of the past, from the ancient Greek physician Hippocrates, to the warriors of Sparta and beyond. It's called intermittent fasting, and it will totally revolutionize the way you live, look, feel, and think!

While it has long been forgotten, it has recently been rediscovered and is quickly becoming one of the most popular ways to burn fat, boost your mind, heal your body, fight depression, and give yourself the gift of longevity.

First things first: What exactly is intermittent fasting? Intermittent fasting (or IF) is basically a term for a way to lose weight, improve your health, mind, mood, and longevity, by regularly cycling between periods of fasting and periods of non-fasting (often called "feeding"). People often confuse intermittent fasting with calorie restriction diets but while IF gives you all of the health and weight loss benefits of calorie restriction, it does so without saddling you with the enormous cravings, crippling fatigue, and constant calorie counting that are part of the calorie restriction way of eating.

Another thing that sets IF apart from other nutrition plans is that is quite simply NOT a diet at all. Diets are tough to stick to, physically, mentally, and emotionally grueling, and very often quite boring, limited, and restrictive. IF is the exact opposite—while you have to dramatically cut your caloric intake, it's only for a very short period of time. The rest of the time, you can really eat as you normally do, without worrying about measuring grams, calories, and portions. IF is different because it is a natural way of living for the human body. We've always gone through periods of abundant food supply, often followed by times where food was scarcer, so our bodies are already pros at cycling between fasting and eating. Occasionally going extended periods without taking in any calories is not only an ability that our bodies were made with, it turns out it's also a fantastic mechanism for achieving everything from weight loss to a longer life.

Fasting Is Not Unfamiliar Territory: Did you know that you're already a seasoned faster? You may not realize it but every time you head to bed, you're practicing intermittent fasting, simply by going to sleep!

Every minute from the last meal you eat at night all the way up until your first meal of the next day makes up a long stretch of time in which you are not eating—basically this is your fasting period. The stretch of time from your first meal all the way up until the last meal you eat that day makes up your feeding period. This is a perfect example of the principles of intermittent fasting. So if you usually eat your dinner at about 9 PM and you don't eat anything else until breakfast at about 9 AM, you're actually completing a pretty impressive 12 hour fast, without even thinking about it. So, as you can you see, intermittent fasting is not some radical, unknown new diet. It's actually the way we as a species have always lived. The only difference is that now science is finally catching up. Clinical research has proved that IF is not simply something you should do when food or the opportunity to eat isn't available, but rather a vital part of maintaining health and keeping physically, mentally, and emotionally fit and sound.

While people have fasted for thousands of years in an effort to rebalance their bodies and reinvigorate themselves, new studies are showing us that intermittent fasting may be the cure to many of the ills that come with our hectic, over-fed, under-nourished, and unhealthy modern lifestyle.

We now have tons of data backing up what ancient fasters always knew: aside from sleep, fasting may be the single most important, most revitalizing, most intensely repairing activity you can do for your body and mind.

Why Fast? The Almost-Too-Good-To Be-True Benefits of Intermittent Fasting:

When IF is carried out properly, it can do a myriad of truly amazing things for literally every part of you.

When we talk about what fasting intermittently helps you to achieve, it really sounds like everyone's body and brain wish-list. IF's benefits include lowering and controlling your blood sugar levels, helping you to lose weight, lowering your cholesterol, giving you boundless energy, pumping up your brain's powers, and even extending the length of your life!

With effects like these, it's no wonder that IF has become one of the most popular eating movements recently, and as more and more people see real results, often losing stubborn weight they've been carrying around for years or totally reversing lifelong chronic diseases, it's set to become even more popular.

While this book goes in-depth to show you just how IF can totally change the way you look, feel, and function in later chapters, let's take a moment right now to look at some of the astonishing effects that IF can have on your body, mind and life:

IF helps you burn body fat and lose serious weight:

This is probably intermittent fasting's most well-known benefit and since a large portion of the droves of people rushing to try this way of eating are doing so in order to achieve weight loss, it's a good thing that IF has been proven to be an exceptional way to burn fat and regulate hormones while gaining muscle. And surprisingly, it works far better than simply restricting calories!

IF changes the way your body's cells, hormones, and genes function:

Who knew that missing a meal could do so much good? Every time someone practicing IF doesn't eat for an extended period, a couple of really interesting things start to happen: including cell repair, the balancing of hormone levels, such as insulin, and the activation of protective gene mechanisms that help you to become and stay healthy for longer. The body basically uses the opportunity to go about making necessary fixes and recalibrating itself.

IF can fend off type 2 diabetes, drastically improve insulin sensitivity, and reduce insulin resistance:

This critical property of intermittent fasting could be the cure to one of the most deadly chronic diseases in the world. Type 2 diabetes has become far too common and because researchers now believe that the cause may be found in the way we ramp up our blood sugar levels by taking in calories beyond our bodies' actual physiological needs, fasting may prove to be a much better way to eliminate diabetes than medication and other conventional therapies.

IF can super-charge your brain:

Yes, this is true. In many cultures around the world, restricting the amount of food you take in while studying has always been considered an important method to power up the brain cells and improve memory, and we now know that is EXACTLY what intermittent fasting does. We've always known that what you do to your body is what you do to your brain. Animal studies have shown us that if you want to get back your ability to learn, remember, and even regulate your moods, IF really is the way to go.

IF is a powerful inflammation soother and can also kick oxidative stress out of your body:

If you asked any aging specialist to name two of the biggest factors in the aging process, chances are that he or she would likely point to oxidative stress and inflammation. Both of these processes speed up aging by damaging tissues and cells, and setting off unwanted chain reactions within the body and mind. While these processes are pretty much an unavoidable part of living, the good news is that fasting intermittently can ward off their worst effects while also enhancing your body's ability to deal with them, leaving you looking, feeling, and functioning youthfully for far longer!

IF clears out the backlog of damaged and dysfunctional materials inside your body:

When it comes to cleaning up your body and brain form the inside, it turns out that fasting is your friend. Every time we fast, it gives the cells in our bodies the chance to start a self-cleaning process called "autophagy" that allows for damaged and non-functioning proteins and toxic buildup to be eliminated. There's plenty of proof that this process helps to prevent serious diseases, improves our overall system, and keeps us feeling fit

IF has proven heart-healing abilities:

Want to ward off one of the world's top killers? Well, fasting intermittently for even a brief period of time is an excellent way to fight off heart disease. With its ability to lower dangerously high triglyceride levels while bringing up good HDL cholesterol levels, and with its potent anti-inflammatory benefits, adding just a few days of intermittent fasting to your regular eating plan is a surefire way to protect your cardiovascular health, both now and into the future.

IF might be the cancer-cure doctors have been seeking for so long:

That's right- intermittent fasting is so effective at reducing the risk of cancer and putting your body into the best possible position to halt uncontrolled cell growth that researchers are asking the FDA to approve it as a recognized cancer treatment. In addition to this, IF may also hold the key to helping patients cope with chemotherapy.

IF adds years to your lifespan:

With all of the benefits listed above, it's no wonder that intermittent fasting has also been found to help a variety of living organisms add years to their lives and live well past their "normal" lifespan. But it doesn't stop there. Unlike other tested longevity enhancing methods, IF has the ability not only to help extend life, but to make you healthier, more vital, and more mentally sharp, even in old age.

Eating Is Not An All-Day Buffet And Fasting Is Not Starvation

Looking at this long list of benefits, it's hard to believe that something so simple, non-invasive, and absolutely free could heal and protect so many functions of your body and mind. Still, even though most people are completely bowled over by IF's reputation, there's one thing that often keeps them from committing to giving it a shot: the fasting part.

We've been conditioned to believe that we can go anywhere and feel anything but hungry. Hunger has been given a seriously bad name by the major snack food and fast food companies. With ads for food confronting us everywhere, from the roadside to the internet, it can seem like "fasting" is far too daunting a prospect to even try. That's because we've been brainwashed into believing that if we miss even one single meal, we're seriously harming our bodies.

The truth, of course, is the exact opposite. We human beings were never *made* to eat continually all day, every day. Eating is an incredibly complex and energy consuming process, and each time you digest food, you are utilizing a combination of your brain, your hormones, nerves, blood, internal bacteria, and all of the organs in your digestive system. So it's no wonder that giving yourself a short periodical break from constant eating frees up your body to heal itself, restores your energy, mood, mental acuity, and just generally does wonders for your well-being.

Don't let yourself get sucked into the myth that frequent eating is healthy. It doesn't matter whether you're plowing through a bag of potato chips or nibbling on bunches of kale, if you're eating too often throughout the day, you are absolutely *killing your body*! The number one question I'm asked by those to whom I recommend an intermittent fasting protocol is "But won't I starve?" The truth is that fasting is NOT starving! "Starving" often means going without food forcibly, usually for extremely extended periods of time. It's an uncomfortable, often painful experience. "Fasting", on the other hand, is simply reducing your food intake or going without food for a limited period of time. Those who practice it will tell you that it feels great, as well as providing a roster of unbelievable benefits.

Genetically, we were always made to fast. Humans have an in-built ability to go for stretches of time without eating, and when we do, it kicks into gear ingrained mechanisms that help us to survive these times by boosting our physical and mental functions. Saying that we need to always have a quick snack on hand in order to stay energetic and healthy is not only wrong, it totally ignores our long and very healthy history of eating intermittently as a species. And most importantly, any food limiting or abstinence on an IF plan is temporary. I always tell wary individuals that fasting is not forever, but its great effects really are. Once they understand this and get started, they never look back!

Who Can Benefit From Intermittent Fasting?

Because fasting is an ingrained habit for human beings, and because our bodies and minds are hardwired to be able not only to *survive* during periods of low food supply but to actually *thrive* and do better than when we're eating normally, intermittent fasting is a wonderful weight loss treatment and healing therapy for almost everyone. There are however, some important exceptions to keep in mind.

Pregnancy and Fasting:

I do not ever recommend that pregnant women fast. That's because if you're pregnant, your body is already occupied with a very important and complex job. You're supporting the growth of another being, and you really are "eating for two", so any undue stressors that may arise from fasting intermittently just aren't a great idea during those tricky nine months.

While tests have been inconclusive so far on the safety of fasting while pregnant, I advise that you err on the side of caution on this one and postpone fasting for later.

Diabetes and Fasting:

When it comes to those with a chronic illness such as diabetes, it's always important to get your doctor's advice before proceeding with any new eating plan. With that said, though, I'd like to differentiate here between type 1 and type 2 diabetes. Many type 2 diabetics have found success in controlling and even healing their condition through carefully controlled intermittent fasting. I go into the scientific evidence on IF's positive effects on diabetes later in this book.

However, with type 1 diabetes, intermittent fasting is NOT recommended, and could cause serious complications, such as diabetic ketoacidosis. For this reason, I urge all diabetics to speak with their doctors about fasting before attempting it, but I also really want to stress that it's not at all advisable for type 1 diabetics to fast intermittently, unless advised otherwise by their healthcare provider.

Growing Children and Teenagers and Fasting:

When the body is actively growing and developing as it is in childhood and early adulthood, it's vital that you support it by feeding it a broad variety of nutrients in ample amounts. Also, because intermittent fasting actively shifts hormonal production and secretion, it's not recommended for teenagers, as it may impact the hormonal changes already happening during this stage of their development.

Other than these exceptions, the vast majority of people will likely benefit incredibly from fasting intermittently, and will be able to access wonderful effects, ranging from efficient fat burning and higher energy levels, to a clearer mind and a healthier, longer life!

The list above of IF's amazing effects is by no means exhaustive and. Each person who tries IF for themselves finds that it affects them positively in ways that they never expected, so as you start on this healing journey, you'll definitely see IF recalibrating, rebalancing, and healing your mind and body in ways that haven't even been listed. This is because intermittent fasting is not some unfamiliar new way of dieting—it's your inborn ability, built right into your DNA as a human being. That's why, once you get over any doubts about your ability to sustain it, you'll see just how natural and instinctive it is.

In the next chapter, we'll be looking into stories about famous historical figures who successfully used fasting and intermittent fasting's long and successful history as the number one way to heal and rebuild a strong, fit body and mind that are full of vitality and vigor!

Chapter 2: The History of Intermittent Fasting: An Ancient Cure That Still Works Today!

"Our food should be our medicine. Our medicine should be our food. But to eat when you are sick is to feed your sickness."

Hippocrates, renowned physician of ancient Greece and the "Father of Western Medicine"

I'm going to ask you a deceptively simple question: When was the last time you were hungry? If your answer was a couple of hours after breakfast this morning or this afternoon, when the effects of lunch started to wear off, then you, like the vast majority of people, have never been truly hungry.

If you noticed, I asked—when was the last time you *were* hungry, instead of when was the last time you *felt* hungry.

That one word makes all the difference, because in our modern times, most of us constantly *feel* hungry but that doesn't mean that we actually *are* hungry.

With the abundance of easily available food, high calorie beverages, and constant snacking between meals, it's been generations since we've actually felt real hunger.

 So what's wrong with that, you may ask? After all, isn't one of the benefits of modern life the fact that food is always conveniently available? One look around you and you'll have the answer to that question. Today a whopping 2.1 billion people worldwide are obese, that's a shocking 30 % of the world's population. And it's not all about the weight. The deadly side effects of our modern "eat all day, everyday" lifestyle are starting to explode globally, with nearly 2 million deaths from diabetes every year, 17.3 million deaths from cardiovascular disease annually, and more than 10 different types of some of the most fatal cancers being linked to obesity! And that's just the body—when we look at the effects of all that eating on our brains, the picture becomes even more disturbing.

While for years, researchers were mystified about the cause of rapidly rising rates of degenerative diseases of the mind such as Alzheimer's and Parkinson's, they have now established a strong link between weight gain and the development of these and all types of dementia. In addition to that, we now know that certain areas of the brain actually shrink when we become overweight, causing us to have poor memory, sharply decreased learning ability, and a lack of good judgment.

Even worse, the myth that we are now a population of "fat and happy" people has been well and truly debunked. Research shows that the spiking levels of blood sugar and the poor insulin responses that we have been cultivating with our frequent eating are at the root of the depression epidemic, with 350 million people now estimated to be suffering from some form of clinical depression worldwide! In fact, depression is now the leading cause of disability in the world.

So there you have it: sick, fat, and sad. These three words are the poisoned fruit of our new way of life.

But it wasn't always this way. In the past, we humans lived lives that were completely free of the diseases of so-called "civilization". Obesity, coronary heart disease, type 2 diabetes, and chronic inflammatory illnesses are not and never were part of our destiny as human beings. Instead, we've largely created these problems for ourselves by willfully forgetting the ancient knowledge of that once kept us fit, fast, and free from sickness. It's a secret that has been passed down from philosophers, to physicians, but it's also something the common man or woman used to know. This knowledge exists in certain societies even today, but is only used in the case of extreme illness. It's been written about for centuries, used for thousands of years, and is simple, powerful and intensely healing. So why is it still a secret?

The answer is because, this knowledge is absolutely free. You don't have to buy any products, take any pills or get a prescription. You don't need a doctor to apply it for you and you don't need a trainer to teach it to you. The fact is that unlike the many other so-called health secrets out there on the market today, nobody profits from this financially. So in this age of huge conglomerates and highly monetized medicine, it's really no wonder that the secret of intermittent fasting is being closely held, rather than spread.

It's something that anyone, anywhere can do, naturally, easily and 100% on their own! It simply entails abstaining from food for a limited period of time, followed by eating normally. That's it! It's that easy, but don't let the simplicity fool you. Intermittent fasting may be the most powerful weapon our bodies and brains have against the onslaught of deadly chronic conditions that have left us ill, overweight, and physically and mentally broken.

Fasting, in and of itself, is such an ingrained, instinctive behavior that it is done not only by humans but even by other mammals. In fact, when almost any type of mammal becomes sick, it immediately turns away from food. Instead, the animal will find a source of water and will only drink water until they are healed. They will then return to eating normally.

If you have a pet dog, then you've probably seen this firsthand. Even the slightest level of illness is enough to make your dog absolutely refuse to feed. It's part of a natural protective response because animals know instinctively that while eating will often cause the problem to get worse, abstaining from food for a short period will help their bodies rebalance and fight off whatever illness they're facing. This is a response we humans also used to have but many centuries of dulling our natural reactions have made most of us incapable of remembering and using the wisdom we were born with.

Still, even now, in almost every culture in the world, there remain small traces of the wisdom of fasting intermittently for health. For example, have you ever heard the well-known saying "starve a fever"? This wise maxim is not just an old wives' tale. In fact, it is based on the very real fact that fevers are a sign of out-of-control inflammation, and that eating when experiencing a fever will cause the inflammation to rage for longer, while eliminating food for a short period will actually work to cool the inflammation that is at the root of the problem.

And science now shows us that this is indeed true: A Dutch study proved that fasting while suffering from a high grade fever worked on the immune system to stop the fever in its tracks. This is just one small example of intermittent fasting's intensely curative power. Every time we go without food for an extended period of time, we are literally reconfiguring, cleansing, and rebooting our systems. So, when I asked you above, "When was the last time you were hungry?" what I really meant was "When was the last time you gave your body and mind the incredibly healing gift of hunger?"

Intermittent Fasting In History

Intermittent fasting has a long and rich history rooted in many nations and societies around the globe. It has been used by princes and paupers, noblemen and commoners. But because of its renowned results, it has also been studied and practiced by some of the most well-known thinkers, physicians, and creators of all time. Let's take a brief look at what some of the most famous individuals in history knew about fasting intermittently:

Did you know that Hippocrates, the most famous physician of ancient Greece and a man whose work was so influential that he is acknowledged today as the "Father of Western Medicine", was an avid intermittent faster? Hippocrates advocated fasting in order to heal any form of illness, and he himself would often use intermittent fasting to restore his wellness. Hippocrates was well known for fasting from seven to ten days at a time. He would often prescribe similar fasts to his patients. It is from this great man of medicine that we have one of the most important quotes about fasting in medical history: *"Everyone has a doctor in him; we just have to help him in his work. The natural healing force within each one of us is the greatest force in getting well."*

As a regular intermittent faster, Hippocrates was able to maintain his good health and vibrancy late into his life. He is one of our first examples of the life-extending power of fasting. While some records date his death to be at the age of 90, others show that he lived until the ripe old age of 100!

This natural healing force that Hippocrates spoke of is the innate ability to fast for certain periods of time, allowing us to truly heal our bodies from illness, obesity, fatigue, and aging, and our brains from damage, shrinking, and dysfunction. And Hippocrates wasn't alone in understanding the benefits of fasting. Plato, the famed philosopher, used fasting to sharpen his thought processes, even declaring *"I fast for greater physical and mental efficiency."*

The 2nd century physician and philosopher Galen practiced medicine among the upper classes of Rome and was also the personal physician to Emperor Commodus. Because the Romans of the Emperor's court were known for excessive over-eating, this gave Galen the opportunity to really see up close the dangers of frequent feasting and helped him to understand how fasting could heal and cool the many inflammatory diseases caused by constant eating. Galen often prescribed and used intermittent fasts, and his life and work has contributed immensely to our understanding of healing. Both Galen and Plato lived very long lives, with Galen dying at the age of 87 and Plato dying at the age of 84, reportedly in sound mind and good health. From ancient Greece to medieval times and beyond, we have always known that fasting intermittently can help our bodies and minds to function properly and that it can even add years to our lives.

How Fasting Can Help You Live to Be 100: The Incredible Case of Luigi Cornaro

In 1504, a Venetian nobleman named Luigi Cornaro lay in his bed preparing to die. He was just 40 years old. He was a wealthy, powerful man and had the services of the very best doctors money could buy, but no one could save his life.

He had seen all of the top physicians of Genoa, and all were convinced that his illness was absolutely incurable. One doctor, however, came forward and gave Luigi the simple advice that rescued him from an early death. From questioning and examining Luigi, this doctor was able to recognize the problem. As a rich, young nobleman, Luigi had access to the good life, and that meant unlimited amounts of the finest foods and beverages, non-stop. The doctor told Luigi that if he really wanted to live past 40, he would have to eliminate his habit of frequent, round-the-clock eating. Like all chronic over-feeders, Luigi struggled with the concept of not eating all day, every day but the close proximity of impending death forced him to take his doctor's advice. Very quickly, Luigi went from an overweight, overloaded, jaundiced, and highly inflamed man at the end of his life to a lean, fit, vibrant many who was able to enjoy his life fully. The difference—instead of gorging on the many feasts enjoyed by his peers at the time, Luigi saved his body by re-teaching it how to fast!

For extended periods of time, he allowed himself only 420 grams of food per day, made up of items such as eggs, meat, and fish and vegetable soup, and divided into two separate meals. Luigi's fast was actually very similar to the fast days prescribed on the 5:2 fast that I explain in a later chapter of this book.

He was soon able to leave his bed and begin a brand new life of health and vitality. He maintained these great results until he was 78. At this time, as is so often the case for those who try fasting, his close friends and family members convinced him to give up his long fasts and instead to eat as frequently as he liked. Luigi went back to the kind of non-stop, all day chronic eating that had caused him so much pain decades before, and it wasn't long before he felt the terrible effects. Feeling more ill, weak, fatigued, and heavy than he had for years, Luigi was at the point of death yet again. He was suffering from a raging fever, which medical knowledge now tells us is a primary sign of inflammation.

He knew he had to take drastic action before the effects of his overeating dragged him back to his deathbed. He began to fast again and marvelously, though he was much older than he had been when he first tried fasting at 40, it worked in exactly the same way! Luigi regained his health and vigor and was able to live well past anyone's expectations— even his own. He had always wanted to live to the age of 100, but because of the revitalizing benefits of his long periods of fasting he was able to overshoot that goal, living until the age of 103 and dying peacefully, as he slept in his rocking chair. At the time of his death, Luigi Cornaro had enjoyed a long, rich, and energetic life, free from illness, except on the occasions when he began to eat frequent meals all day with abandon.

Through fasting, Luigi had found the fountain of youth that we all seek so desperately, and had also discovered that not only had fasting made his body more fit, it had also preserved all of his faculties. Up until the day of his death, he was able to hear and see perfectly.

Although he was a centenarian, he never suffered from any senility and possessed an exceptional memory until the very end. In today's world, where we regularly see people developing Alzheimer's and other forms of dementia and memory loss at only 50 years old, Luigi Cornaro's amazing journey to lifelong health is an example to us of how intermittent fasting can powerful treat our bodies, sharpen our minds, and extend our lives!

The Story of Dr. Otto Buchinger: How Fasting Intermittently Saved This Pioneer of Medical Fasting From a Life of Disability

Few stories highlight the healing powers of intermittent fasting like the case of Dr. Otto Buchinger. Dr. Buchinger was a German doctor and a pioneer of utilizing fasting as a medical treatment. Although his father had wanted him to be a lawyer, Buchinger was passionate about studying medicine. After he received a doctorate, he served as a naval doctor during World War I. But soon after achieving his dream, everything came crashing down around him in 1917. In the midst of a promising medical career, Buchinger was hit by a serious illness: infected rheumatism affecting his joints.

The infected rheumatism spread throughout the joints in his body so rapidly that it was only a short while before he found himself completely unable to move. The tragedy-stricken young doctor had no choice but to leave his position. In extreme pain and completely disabled, he searched for a medical solution from doctor after doctor, but found no hope. Finally, when had lost all confidence in conventional treatments, he began to seek alternative treatment options.

This led him to the office of Dr. Riedlin, a physician who was known for using intermittent fasting therapies to heal his patients. Dr. Riedlin examined Buchinger and immediately placed him on a course of fasting. From that moment, the young doctor's life changed. He began to recover rapidly as the fasting treatment cooled, calmed, and eliminated the inflammatory causes of his painful and debilitating condition. Soon, he was able to move around freely again, and he couldn't believe that simply fasting for limited periods could reverse and heal what conventional doctors were unable to treat! He would later write that receiving that fasting treatment saved his life.

It was at this point that Dr. Buchinger became very involved with learning more about the ancient history of fasting and using this knowledge to develop a method of intermittent fasting that could provide patients, who like him had been told their conditions were hopeless, with effective medical fasting treatments. He opened his own fasting medical clinics, where over 250,000 people have benefitted from the same incredible healing that Dr. Buchinger experienced when he tried his first fast. Dr. Buchinger experienced seeing so many patients healed of their ailments through fasting on minimal calories for a limited period that he even called fasting "the operation without surgery"!

According to Buchinger, fasting allows each person to activate the innate self-healing powers within the body. I've seen this to be true in so many cases today, time and time again. No matter how run down or hopeless you think your condition is, once you start this journey to health through intermittent fasting, I can assure you that you WILL see the same benefits that we humans have always gained through this ancient healing practice.

Join me in the following sections, where we'll look at the many different ways to fast intermittently, the benefits of each, and which one is right for you!

Chapter 3: The Classic 5:2 Fast—Eat What You Want For Most Of Your Week And Still See Amazing Results!

After seeing so many people try, struggle, and fail through weight loss gimmick after faddy weight loss gimmick, I don't believe in diets. As I've explained before, intermittent fasting is not a diet. Instead, it's an eating pattern that is all about scheduling and not about constant calorie counting. It's not about pre-packaged shakes and expensive, usually unhealthy "weight loss bars", or ridiculous amounts of exercise that the average working person will never be able to find the time to complete. It's about regaining control of when you eat, instead of relying on outdated ideas about "3 square meals day" or "frequent small meals throughout the day". Most people have spent a lifetime listening to advice from one conflicting diet book after another and are left feeling thoroughly confused and powerless. I wrote this guide to tell you that you are NOT powerless, and that, with intermittent fasting, you can take back control of your weight, health, mood, and mind. Not only that, but you can do it without any fancy equipment or hyped up so-called super foods. At the core of it, all you need is your body and a clock or watch. That's really it!

Now, there are several different ways of doing intermittent fasting. Some ways are clearly better than others, scientifically, and in in my opinion, but before getting into each, I'd like you to know that any type of intermittent fast is much, much better than the typical eating schedule so many of us are on, and also light years better than any of the many diet plans out there.

With that said, I will admit, I do have favorites among the various types, and I also believe that some types don't work as well as others for the vast majority of people. However, I want to include the most popular types of IF in this book so that you can get a clear understanding of each method and make an informed choice about which method works best for you. Additionally, many people start off intermittently fasting by using one method and then gradually switching to another method of IF, until they find what suits their bodies and schedules most.

So in this and following chapters, we'll be looking at the 5:2 fast, the 24 hour Eat Stop Eat Fast and the Warrior fast. These each have differing schedules, nutritional recommendations, and rules, but they can all be used as forms of intermittent fasting, and each delivers the intensive fat burning, inflammation quenching, and mind clearing results that are part and parcel of IF.

Let's get started!

The 5:2 Fast: How to Lose Weight While Eating What You Want Most of the Time!

First, we have the classic 5:2 fast, also known as "the two day fast". This type of intermittent fasting is more widely recognized than other varieties. Its name comes from its distinctive fasting and feeding cycle. On the 5:2, you basically eat as you always do for five days of the week, while "fasting" by reducing your caloric intake to about 500 calories for women and 600 calories for men for two days of the week.

An important point to note is that you should never fast on two consecutive days of the week. So for instance, if you've chosen a Monday as your first fast day, you should follow it up with normal eating on Tuesday and choose one of the remaining days of the week for your second day of fasting. On the 5:2 fast, an average man's week may look like fasting by consuming only 600 calories in food and beverages on Monday, eating his usual 2500 calories worth of meals on Tuesday, fasting again on 600 calories on Wednesday and then spending Thursday through Sunday eating his usual 2500 calories every day. This is perhaps what makes this type of fasting so popular. It's not like a diet that tells you to restrict or severely reduce your calorie intake every day of the week. Instead, it's an eating strategy that allows you to eat as you always have for five out of seven of the days of the week, and only requires you to restrict your calories for two days of the week. Many people love the freedom this gives them, allowing them to make a sacrifice for a short time and enjoy the reward of being able to eat normally for the remainder of the time. Sounds good, right? But does it work?

To answer that, let's go into the kind of results the 5:2 fast produces.

Benefits of The 5:2 Fast

On the two days when you are eating 500-600 calories a day, your body realizes it's not getting enough fuel from meals, so what does it do? First, it uses up all the emergency glycogen stored in your liver, and when that runs out, it gets busy burning off your fat reserves for energy instead. This obviously leads to weight loss, because your stored up fat becomes your body's only source of fuel.

But how can this be, considering that you'll be eating normally on the remaining 5 days of the week? Well, here's the really exciting part of the 5:2 fast.

Studies done by Valter Longo, a biologist at the University of Southern California, show that in animal testing, when test subjects fast for limited periods and binge on food when they aren't fasting, they STILL manage to lose weight! And this is exactly what people who go on the 5:2 fast find—that despite making up for the days they fasted by eating a large amount on non-fast days, they are actually dropping pounds and feeling better. So basically, if the 5:2 fast had a motto, it would be, "Lose weight while eating the same amount of food."

But before you jump into this fast wholeheartedly, keep this in mind: just because you'll still lose weight if you eat only 500-600 calories for a couple of days and binge on fast-food for the rest of the week doesn't mean that it's recommended. And most people aren't turning to this type of intermittent fasting because they want to eat unlimited amounts of junk food. Instead, this fast is so popular because it allows people to live without the constant restrictions of dieting and gives them the opportunity to spend most of their week eating until they are completely satisfied, rather than spending all seven days of the week on a highly restrictive, unrealistic diet that leaves them hungry, tired, miserable, and struggling to see results.

And there's one other amazing effect of fasting the 5:2 way—appetite suppression! After only a couple of weeks on this type of fast, people report that although they thought they'd be absolutely ravenous on their non-fasting days, they actually have a more controlled appetite, and their cravings for sugary, carb-laden foods are almost completely eliminated. And this isn't just a momentary change. Results show that those who have fasted intermittently are able to avoid hunger pangs and cravings for junk food long after their initial fasting period. It appears that the 5:2 fast works on your mind and body to produce stronger feelings of satiety and by increasing your insulin sensitivity, it allows you to be set free from the massive cravings for carbs and sugary snacks that are at the root of why so many diets fail.

If you're one of the many people who are more than happy to tough it out with a couple of low calorie days every week, in order to be free from restrictions on the other five days of your week, this plan is perfect for you. However, you may find it difficult to adjust to living on 500-600 calories initially, and you may want to ease into the 5:2 fast by gradually decreasing the number of calories you eat on fast days. Many people have found success with limiting themselves to 800 calories at first and then going even lower until they feel comfortable fasting at 500-600 calories.

How Do I Split Up My Meals On Fast Days On the 5:2 Fast?

As you know, all intermittent fasting methods are centered on timing, so *when* you choose to ingest your 500-600 calories on fasting days is very important. I often advise people starting out on this type of fast to split their calories into two meals because trying to space out such a small number of calories throughout several meals will only leave you feeling unsatisfied and may end up triggering your hunger rather than satiating it. The best way to achieve this is to have a mid-day meal at about 12 noon that uses up half of your calories and then three to four hours before your normal bedtime, eat the second half of your calories. So if you're on the 600 calorie plan, this would mean a lunch that contains 300 calories and an early dinner that comes in at another 300 calories. Your lunch meal will give you the fuel to get through your day normally and your early dinner meal will prevent you from suffering late night hunger and sleeplessness.

You can also supplement these main meals with no-calorie beverages such as coffee, black tea, green tea, and herbal teas, as well as chewing a few sticks of sugar–free gum to keep your mouth occupied and help pass the time. In the case that your main meals come in a little bit under your allowed calorie count, feel free to use these extra calories to add a splash of milk or small spoon of honey to your coffee or tea.

For reasons based on your body's natural pattern of secreting insulin which I'll explain in depth in the following chapters, I do not ever recommend you eating breakfast as one of your fast day meals. You'll find yourself feeling much fuller and stronger if you split your calorie intake between lunch and dinner, and you'll also be prolonging the stretch between meals, allowing you to burn even more fat.

So What Makes The 5:2 Fast Different From Low Calorie Diets?

Well, the most important difference is that with 5:2, you are only eating low calorie meals for two days instead of every day of the week. This makes it much easier to stick with and also, surprisingly, those who fast on only two days actually show more weight loss than those who restrict their calories every day!

Another difference is in the fact that there are no "forbidden foods" on the 5:2 fast, and no calorie counting for the majority of your week. When you are on a non-fast day, you're encouraged to eat as you normally do.

As I mentioned, this doesn't necessarily mean heading straight for your nearest fast-food outlet, but it does mean having a lot more freedom and flexibility. On the 5:2 fast, you can easily go out to dinner with friends on a non-fast day, ditch the calorie counting, and forget about portion sizes. As long as you're sure to eat within your guidelines for the two fasting days, the non-fasting days are yours to enjoy pretty much as you please. This is why people find 5:2 so much more effective than other weight loss plans, and why they adopt it as a way of life that provides lasting results rather than just a temporary fix.

My Top Tips For A Successful 5:2 Fast:

Tip #1: Think Protein and Plants On 5:2 fast Days

While it is indeed possible to fast on 500 calories of pure carbs, it's certainly not a good idea and would end up sabotaging your long term weight loss and health by spiking massive insulin releases. I recommend that you think mostly "Protein and Plants" when it comes to the meals you have on your fast days. This way, you'll feel nourished, experience lower levels of hunger, and you'll be maximizing the powerful health and weight loss benefits of your fast!

Tip # 2: Stay Hydrated I mention this throughout this book because it's one of the most important things you can do to make your fasting efforts really pay off. Don't sabotage your fast by allowing yourself to become dehydrated. Instead, amp up your fat burning metabolism and keep yourself safe, energetic, and focused by drinking at least eight glasses or two liters of water per day on fast days. If you'll be outdoors or doing heavy lifting, add a little more to be on the safe side.

Tip # 3: Make It Easier on Yourself By Preparing In Advance Unlike the other fasting methods, because you'll be consuming a certain amount of calories on your 5:2 fast days, give yourself the best shot at success by making sure you've got meals and beverages prepped ahead of time. This way, there'll be no room for calorie mistakes or temptations causing your fast to come to a grinding halt.

Tip # 4: Spice It Up Although you only have a very small amount of calories to play with on your fast days, you can still make really satisfying meals by adding no or low calorie flavors, like spices or a squeeze of lemon. You'll be surprised at how much more you enjoy your small meal when it has a little spice and zing added to it!

Tip # 5: Don't Lose Heart on Fast Days It can be a little harder to stick with a 5:2 fast because you're eating small amounts of food which are often just enough to spark your appetite but not enough to actually fill you up. Take a deep breath and realize that hunger pangs are a reminder that your body is about to go into all of the wonderful processes that speed up cell repair, massively increase weight loss, slow down the aging process, heal diabetes and other chronic illnesses, and prevent cancer. Hunger pangs are letting you know you are on the right track: keep going and remember, you have five fast-free days to look forward to!

If you're looking for a shorter, more targeted way to fast, read on to the next chapter, where we'll explore a type of intermittent fasting that gives you results in just 24 hours!

Chapter 4: The 24 Hour Fast: "Eat Stop Eat" Your Way To A Better Body, With As Little As One Fast Day!

While the 5:2 fast has worked wonders for many people, there are still some who find the need to stay within a set caloric limit on fast days a major drawback of the plan.

If you're looking or a way to lose weight, retain muscle, and maintain high levels of energy, without having to count calories or restrict food, then I recommend the "Eat Stop Eat" way of fasting, otherwise known as the 24 hour fast. This revolutionary way of intermittently fasting provides those who use it with a very simple plan: you fast for an entire 24 hour period, once or twice a week, depending on your weight loss goals and how quickly you'd like to drop the pounds.

Unlike the 5:2 fasting method, with Eat Stop Eat, no calories are consumed during this 24 hour fast period, making it a more powerful, focused type of intermittent fasting. However, you are still able to drink plenty of non-calorie beverages like coffee, black tea, and green and herbal teas. Most individuals who follow this fasting method prefer to fast from 6 pm the previous night until 6 pm the next evening—making it a full 24 hours without caloric intake. However, there's plenty of room to play around with the times, as long as you make sure to eat your last meal at least three hours before your bedtime, to ensure proper metabolism and health. After the 24 hour fast period is over, you simply go back to eating as normal!

In fact, the creator of this fast plan actually advises you to act as if you haven't fasted at all. You don't reduce your caloric intake, restrict, or change your usual eating habits at all. And yet, with just one or two fast days a week, you still see amazing results that many Eat Stop Eat fasters say far outstrips the weight loss they've achieved on low calorie diet plans.

A word of caution, though—once fasters see the accelerated weight loss that this type of intermittent fasting produces, they're often tempted to do back to back fasts, or pack in more than two fasts a week. Eat Stop Eat guidelines are very clear in this regard: never wear out your system and your metabolism by fasting on two consecutive days, and never do more than two fasts in a seven day period. Not only is this counter-productive, as it can send distress signals to your body that actually end up slowing your fat burning response down, it's also unnecessary, because even a one day a week 24 hour fast is enough to create a caloric deficit of 10% and leave you much slimmer and fitter in the process.

So How Does It Work?

Eat Stop Eat primarily works for two reasons: one is the undeniable fact that removing one or two days' worth of eating from your week is going to end up cutting quite a lot of caloric intake from your overall consumption. Let's say for instance that you normally eat 2500 calories per day. That would be 17,500 calories in 7 days. However, with the Eat Stop Eat intermittent fasting method, you'd be removing up to two days of eating from your week, effectively cutting 5000 calories from your week's consumption, leaving you with only 12,500. Because it's commonly accepted that you need to cut 3,500 calories in order to lose one pound of weight, this alone would be enough to see you losing nearly one and a half pounds of weight a week. However, that's not really the whole story.

The majority of fasters on the Eat Stop Eat method report losing more weight than merely one and a half pounds per week, with some seeing weight loss of up to 2-3 pounds weekly, even though they're only reducing 5000 calories from their weekly total. Granted, in the first weeks, a large proportion of this is actually water weight stored up due to tissue inflammation, but as the fast begins to reduce systemic inflammation, real weight is also lost.

Additionally, they don't experience the massive muscle loss that most dieters go through when losing weight. Instead, many Eat Stop Eat fasters find that when they exercise, they gain and retain muscle mass more easily following their fasting periods. So if the answer isn't purely in reduction of caloric intake, then what's behind the enhanced fat loss and muscle mass gain that this method provides?

This brings us to the second reason that Eat Stop Eat and all intermittent fasting methods work so well, better, in most cases, than even the strictest diets. Fasting for a long stretch of time (anywhere from 16 to 24 hours) brings about physiological shifts in our bodies that appear to hit the reset button on all of our functions, causing our body to work more smoothly, efficiently, and effectively.

When you do an Eat Stop Eat 24 hour fast, your body first burns off all the glucose available from previous meals, and then gets through the glycogen stored within your liver. Then, with all of the easy fuel gone, it realizes it's going to need to keep running and starts to burn fat, producing ketones, a source of energy only produced when you aren't constantly refueling yourself with glucose-producing foods as its source of energy. What happens next is the key to the fat loss that happens when you fast intermittently: because of a lack of food, your body begins to focus only on burning fat, without touching your muscles. This means you can lose large amounts of weight without in any way compromising your existing muscle mass, leaving you not only thinner but also leaner and fitter.

Additionally, a review published in the American Journal of Clinical Nutrition found that the type of alternate day fasting that Eat Stop Eat is founded on led to a significantly decreased risk of chronic disease. Because chronic diseases are largely inflammatory at their root, these results clearly show the link between Eat Stop Eat fasting and a lower level of inflammation. This inflammation cooling effect may also have a lot to do with the weight loss benefits provided by Eat Stop Eat, as we know that most who are suffering from inflammatory conditions find stubborn weight gain to be one of the most persistent symptoms of their illness.

Finally, Eat Stop Eat fasting has a deeply cleansing effect on the body, on a cellular level. This type of cellular cleansing produces a highly detoxifying response, clearing out a whole backlog of built-up debris and toxins from deep within the cells and allowing the body to re-establish a healthy metabolism, now that it is free from the struggle of dealing with these toxic materials.

So, as you see, it's not really all just about calories in, calories out. And when it comes to weight loss on the typical version of Eat Stop Eat method of fasting, it's also not about cutting any particular food group out of your life. The fast's creator insists that you can really eat just about anything on your non-fasting days, which make up the majority of your week. In fact, people have been known to eat even high carb foods that are usually banned on diets, such as cake or pizza, and still lose weight. However, this fast method doesn't allow for an all-out binge, so if you want pizza, you can have a couple of slices without worrying but you can't inhale the whole pie.

As long as you eat responsibly and don't try to "reward" yourself for the calories you lost on the fast days by excessively overeating on your non-fast days, you will see steady weight loss on this plan. I recommend this fast method if you are the type of person who prefers to do a once or twice a week fast, eat normally throughout the rest of the week, never count calories, and still see consistent fat loss. However, it is more difficult to pull off than the previously discussed 5:2 method because you don't have that 500 to 600 calorie cushion on fast days that allows you to feel more satiated. For some, however, that's more of a solution than a problem.

Regular Eat Stop Eat fasters discover that not eating at all on fast days basically switches off their appetites and awareness of food, and they claim that eating the meager calories allowed on the 5:2 fast days only serves to make them feel more hungry and less able to stick with the full day fast.

And here's where personal experimentation really counts. Each method of intermittent fasting provides the proven benefits of fasting, but each also has its own rules and restrictions. I always counsel anyone who comes to me seeking to do an intermittent fast to try each of the methods I explain in this book out before selecting just one method. This is because everyone's metabolism, hunger threshold, and schedule differs, and finding the perfect fit for your body and lifestyle just isn't possible without a little willingness to experiment.

My Top Tips For A Successful Eat Stop Eat Fast:

Tip# 1: Hone Your Self Control By Going Slowly I always recommend a gradual approach to intermittent fasting because it's vital that you don't shock yourself by taking on too much at once. People who have no experience with missing meals or who have practiced the "eat 6 small, frequent meals throughout the day" method of nutrition for many years will find it extremely difficult to suddenly go an entire 24 hours without food. I've seen very determined, focused individuals miss out on what really is one of the most powerful ways to lose weight and get healthy, simply because they tried to do too much at once and ended up so uncomfortable with the experience of suddenly fasting that they lost the motivation to continue. Our bodies and our minds both operate very much on habit, so no matter how eager you are to get started, surprising your system with a cold-turkey 24 hour fast is not going to produce the long term results you want. My remedy: I like to advise a regimen in which individuals begin by reducing the frequency of eating and cutting a substantial but not uncomfortable amount of calories from their daily meals. If you usually eat three meals per day, totaling 2500 calories, I'd have you reduce this down to two meals totaling 900 calories per day for a couple of days, then a single meal totaling 700 calories for another few days, then a single meal totaling 500 calories per day. After this, you're ready to try out a full 24 hour fast, because your body and mind have both begun to acclimate to the idea of eating less frequently and running efficiently on far fewer calories.

If you find it too difficult to hit the 24 hour mark without food on your first try, don't worry. Simply try to go as long as possible without eating, and break your fast when the wait becomes truly unbearable. On your following attempts, try to stretch the fasting period even further and you may find yourself fasting a full 24 hours before you know it.

Tip # 2: Remember To Eat Responsibly Although the Eat Stop Eat fast doesn't have any forbidden foods or any caloric limits, if you're doing this fast for weight loss or health, nutritional common sense still applies.

What that means for most fasters is that you can eat a reasonable amount of the treats you always enjoy, but that fasting doesn't give you more leeway to overindulge than usual. The typical version of Eat Stop Eat doesn't set any limits for carbohydrates, but does require you to eat anywhere from 20 to 30 grams of high-quality protein every four to five hours, in order to achieve a daily protein total of 100 grams.

However, if you're using this fasting method to lose a large amount of weight, or you'd like to get better blood sugar control, I recommend mixing Eat Stop Eat's 24 hour fasts with a moderate to low carb eating plan, so that you can really reap great results. The added bonus is that even though you're slashing carbs, you're still not cutting calories or reducing portions. During non-fast days, feel free to feast until you're fully satisfied on high protein, high fat and low carb foods, and don't worry about measuring or counting anything, and I guarantee you'll see the weight coming off naturally as your blood sugar levels even out.

Just to give you a clear idea of what this entails, I'd like to explain the difference between eating normally on an Eat Stop Eat fast, versus eating for enhanced weight loss and better blood sugar control on an Eat Stop Eat fast. Let's examine this briefly below:

Sample Plan & Schedule: Eating Normally on An Eat Stop Eat Fast

The Day Before Fasting Day: Last meal is eaten at 8 PM. No snacks or caloric beverages are consumed after this time.

The Fasting Day: No foods or caloric beverages are consumed throughout the day. Calorie-free beverages such as coffee, and black, green, and herbal teas are permitted. At 8 PM, 24 hours later, the fast is broken with any kind of meal you choose, in any amount that satisfies you fully, and without any need to measure caloric content.

The Following Non-Fasting Day: You eat as usual, again, without worrying about caloric content, carb or fat content or amount, but also keeping in mind both the need to eat up to 100 grams of protein per day, and the need to eat neither less nor more food than usual.

Sample Plan & Schedule: Eating For Enhanced Weight Loss and Better Blood Sugar Control on An Eat Stop Eat Fast

The Day Before Fasting Day: High protein, high fat, low carb last meal is eaten at 8 PM. An ideal meal would be a large portion of beef, chicken, or fish, a small portion of non-starchy, low Glycemic Index vegetables, and an added portion of fat from grass-fed butter, coconut oil, or other pure fat sources. No sugary beverages or snacks are consumed with this meal, and no snacks or caloric beverages are consumed after this time.

The Fasting Day: No foods or caloric beverages are consumed throughout the day. Calorie-free beverages such as coffee, and black, green, and herbal teas are permitted. At 8 PM, 24 hours later, the fast is broken with another high protein, high fat, low carb meal of your choice, in any amount that satisfies you fully, and without any need to measure caloric content.

The Following Non-Fasting Day: You eat as usual, again, without worrying about caloric content or amount, but also keeping in mind the need to limit foods and beverages that are high in carbohydrates or sugar. With this version of the Eat Stop Eat fast, you do not need to worry about eating the same amount as always. Instead, because you're eating a drastically lower amount of carbohydrates, you have the ability to eat larger portions than you usually do, and still achieve both weight loss and better blood sugar control.

As you can see, both plans are remarkably similar and only differ in two ways: with the normal eating plan, you are able to eat any type of food you usually consume, within a reasonable amount. With the high fat, high protein, and low carb plan, you don't have to worry about eating the amount you always eat, and can exceed this if you're hungry. But you do need to pay attention to cutting carbs, especially when first breaking your fast. The results of both plans are also similar, but those who use the low carb version of this fast do find that they lose weight more easily and quickly, and that they see an even more intense improvement in their energy levels and a major drop in their blood sugar levels.

So who would benefit from these plans? I recommend the normal Eat Stop Eat fast plan if you want to simply lose weight, rebalance your energy, and improve your overall general health. If you need to lose a larger amount of weight, have specific chronic inflammatory illnesses including type 2 diabetes, or various conditions such as rheumatoid arthritis, arteriosclerosis, lupus, IBD, Hashimoto's, and any other autoimmune disorders, I strongly recommend opting for the second, high fat, low carb version of this fast.

That's because all of the benefits of Eat Stop Eat are heightened and improved by adding a low carb focus to your eating and also because the added fat and the avoidance of carbohydrates allows you to cool your inflammation levels and protect your central nervous systems through lowering blood sugar WHILE you're in the midst of a serious inflammatory illness. Many people feel that they won't be able to handle a fast during the toughest points of their conditions but adding carb-restriction or elimination to your fast can actually help you to heal faster and more thoroughly.

Tip # 3: Stay Hydrated I can never overstate the importance of staying hydrated while doing any of these intermittent fast methods, but this becomes even more of a critical issue when it comes to the Eat

Stop Eat fast. Because you're eliminating nutrition during your 24 hour fast period, you have a higher likelihood of finding yourself feeling fatigued, weak, and dehydrated on this particular fasting method. Fortunately, beverages are not only allowed on Eat Stop Eat, they are encouraged. Just remember to stick to zero calorie options such as pure water, mineral water, teas, and coffees. A pinch of salt in your drinks can help to rebalance your electrolytes and keep you feeling more alert and less parched throughout the fast period. Always keep a water source on hand and increase the amount you drink if you'll be spending time outside in hot weather or doing any type of physical work. This is extremely important—I've seen far too many people think that just because they're not eating during a fast day, they don't need to worry about drinking either. This often results in dizzy spells, extreme fatigue, crankiness, a lack of concentration, and, in particularly hot weather, it can also end up causing a serious case of heatstroke. In addition to all of that, dehydration has been clinically proven to slow down your metabolism markedly, so not drinking at least eight glasses or two liters of water during your fast can actually undo all of the amazing effects you're trying to achieve through intermittent fasting. Keep yourself protected from illness and exhaustion and make sure you really get all of the weight loss and health benefits you deserve, by staying thoroughly hydrated during and after your fasts.

Now that you've got a handle on the Eat Stop Eat fast, join me in the next chapter for an in-depth look at a modern fast, with its roots in the ancient fasting and feasting patterns of warriors, promising fat-loss, muscle mass, and health results that can't be beat!

Chapter 5: The Warrior Fast: Eat Like An Ancient Warrior For An Unbeatable Body And Brain!

Do you ever wonder how the warriors of the past, such as the Spartans, were able to survive staying on the move all day, doing physically punishing tasks in extreme conditions? Do you long to build that kind of strength and endurance in your own body, to help you deal with the challenges of your own daily life? Are you one of the many people who don't care much for lunch but absolutely *live* for dinner?

If so, I've got just the intermittent fasting method for you: it's called the Warrior fast and it is literally the fasting method that sparked the intermittent fasting craze we are experiencing today!

This type of fasting method is based not necessarily on the modern lifestyles of today but on the ways that tough hardy warriors of the ancient world built strength, stayed lean, and withstood rough, rugged, and sometimes unbearably harsh conditions. This fasting method teaches that if you want a strong lean body you can count on, and a sharp, focused mind, you have to ditch all that you've ever heard about nutrition and begin to eat like a warrior of the ancient world.

The Ethos Behind This Fasting Method:

Like all other intermittent fasting methods, the Warrior fast is based on cycles of fasting and feeding. However, in the case of the Warrior fast, the fasting period far outstrips the feeding period, and the feeding period is much more of a "feasting" period than a regular feeding period. Because this fasting method demands that you fast for 18 or 20 hours per day and that you only eat during a three or four hour window in the evening, it is ideal for those who have a high level of discipline and who also enjoy having their main meal in the evening. This fast was created after deep study into the practices and eating patterns of warriors in the past, and it focuses on the major difference between the average modern human and the tough, disciplined warrior of ancient days. Because humans in the past thrived on periods of under eating and overfeeding, this fast method posits that we should stick as closely to this cycle of intermittent fasting as possible, for optimal health and fitness.

According to this method, the main ingredient that made our predecessors so much more mentally and physically fit is STRESS. Because life in the ancient world was based on the constant struggle for survival, people were exposed to stressors such as cold, heat, exhausting work, and, you guessed it, long periods of hunger on a daily basis. When the comfort of modern-day living took over, it removed almost every source of those stressors, so that now, instead of hunting for food, we simply pick up the phone and order it, and instead of seeking shelter and building fires for warmth, we just press a button for heating. And most importantly, as we go about our days, when we feel even the slightest niggling of hunger (or let's face it, even boredom), we just stroll over to a vending machine and overfeed. This fasting method claims that this has resulted in a population of humans who have all of the genes necessary to be lean, mean, survival machines, but have added layers of fat, weakness, and lack of discipline over the genes, burying them and replacing health and strength with illness and frailty.

Good Stress Versus Bad Stress

This fast method holds that as living beings, we need stress, as long as it's the good kind. All organisms possess a stress-response mechanism that allows them to protect themselves and survive in less than ideal situations. However, without use, over time this mechanism becomes inefficient, ineffective, and leads to health dangers for us. Whenever we experience this type of positive stress, our stress response mechanisms are activated, and we instantly begin to stimulate our nervous system, create muscle tissue, and generally grow stronger, healthier, and leaner. Research into intermittent fasting has shown that repeatedly stressing our bodies and brains with limited periods of fasting does indeed cause each cell within us to switch into high survival gear, allowing it, and therefore us, to function at the very top of our game. This response can often lead to a lowered level of inflammation, higher levels of human growth hormone, and an enhanced metabolism, among other benefits. It works in the same way that physical stress through exercise improves your system.

Now, caloric restriction introduces the same kind of stress to the body, but the main difference is that with constant caloric restriction the body over time begins to feel the strain too keenly and begins to overcompensate by, for instance, slowing the metabolism, or not devoting energy to "non-essential" functions. This means that you are not operating at the top of your game. Instead of stressing the body by introducing caloric restriction, the Warrior fast method cycles fasting periods of up to 18 or 20 hours a day, with periods of eating until totally satisfied.

This fast works by creating a series of temporary fasts that then switch on your stress responders, such as many types of enzymes, stress proteins, and highly anti-inflammatory molecules, which then heal, strengthen, and enhance your mind and body. Studies back this up, showing that fasting throughout the day and eating one large meal aids the health by improving metabolism and weight loss.

How to Follow the Warrior Method of Intermittent Fasting:

To fast in this way, simply schedule in 20 hours of fasting and make sure that this 20 hour period includes all of your sleep time. Next follow this up with 4 hours of overfeeding.

Under-Eating or Fasting?

The fast does allow you to eat small amounts of low calorie, watery and thin foods, if you find it too hard to get through the day without some kind nourishment. The best choices are clear soups, light vegetable juices, coffee, and tea.

If you feel extremely fatigued, a handful of berries or small amounts of sugar-free, all–natural, grass-fed yogurt are also permitted. It's worth noting though, that many choose not to have anything but water and coffee or tea, to maximize benefits. Still, each person's body works differently, and it's important to avoid fatigue, dizziness, and any other side effects of hunger.

Your Feast:

You are advised to eat until completely satisfied in the evening. When you overeat in the evening, your Parasympathetic Nervous System (PNS) is turned on. Your PNS is important in allowing your body to relax, calm down, and recuperate after all of the stresses of the day. It works to improve digestion and helps you utilize the nutrients in your food to repair any damage in your tissues and to grow new, lean muscle.

I don't recommend eating too late in the evening, and I always advise that you eat your last meal at least 3 hours before sleeping. This method of fasting advises you to eat a heavy, large, cooked meal made up of foods that would easily have been recognized in the ancient world—mainly lean meats, wild-caught fish, free-range eggs, fruits, vegetables, root vegetables, legumes, and grass-fed dairy products.

Watch Out For Food Combinations:

On this fast, you are cautioned to avoid many types of food combinations which may inhibit your body's drive towards health. Keep in mind that only vegetables and protein can be mixed with everything. Steer clear of combining grain and fruits, grain and sugar, nuts and fruits, or nuts and sugar.

This fast also follows the idea of eating mainly low GI fruit, such as raspberries, blackberries, strawberries, apples, kiwis, and grapefruits.

Also include the following foods:

- Vegetable, miso, and broth soups
- Plenty of fresh, raw, green vegetables to help the body detoxify
- Grass-fed yogurt and kefir for easily digestible lean protein

But make sure that you avoid highly processed, modern "convenience" foods.

<u>Tip #1: Always Break Your Fast With Fresh Vegetables</u> A large salad dressed with olive oil vinaigrette is ideal, allowing your body to ease into eating and detoxing built-up waste. However, avoid using non-wine based vinegar.

Tip #2: Choose High Quality Proteins

With this fasting method, white fish, beef, poultry, eggs, beans, nuts, and legumes are all recommended. Always eat a salad and vegetables BEFORE you eat your protein when breaking your fast, and ensure that, apart from eggs and nuts, you eat protein-packed items only in the evenings.

Tip#3: Eat Clean, Eat Well, and Don't Count Calories

With the Warrior fast's focus on eating whole, real, and largely organic foods that would have been around thousands of years ago, you don't need to worry about counting calories. One of the main ways that this fast works is by allowing you to overeat in the evening. Therefore, attempting to cut calories and portions will result in less success.

Tip # 4: Guzzle Water

I've said this before and I'll say it again. Please don't attempt to lose water weight by avoiding drinking.

Always keep water with you at all times. Often, fasting can cause you to lose, not just your cravings for food, but your desire to drink water as well. Be ready for this sensation and overcome it with scheduled "drinking" times. The risk of dehydration is even greater when it comes to these longer fasts, so stay vigilant and disciplined about getting your daily hydration in.

Tip # 5: Think About Always Having a Bathroom Handy At First

When you first begin this fasting method, you will notice that you need to urinate more often than usual. This is largely due to the initial water weight that will be flushed out of your system by the elimination of inflammation. Don't worry too much about it, as your urination frequency will gradually slow down and return to normal.

Tip #6: Avoid Hitting The Carbs, If You Can

While carb-cycling can play a role in this fast, it's generally recommended that if you feel fully satisfied on high quality protein, salads, and vegetables, you shouldn't reach for the heavy carbs. You'll certainly still lose weight if you do, but you won't be getting all of the insulin and inflammation lowering benefits you could be getting.

Next, we'll be looking at my personal favorite, a fasting method that combines all of the benefits of intermittent fasting into one potent plan! Trust me, you won't want miss it!

Chapter 6: 16/8:The Secret to Unstoppable Weight Loss, Incredible Health And Intense Energy

If I could only recommend one thing to someone who's struggling with unexplained or stubborn weight gain, feeling sluggish, and suffering from one or more chronic illnesses, it would be these two numbers: 16/8.

That's it! Why? Because those two little numbers stand for a way of eating and living that is so revolutionary, so powerful, and yet so simple that it wouldn't be fair to call it a diet. Allow me to explain. How many times have you gone on diets that promised you amazing weight loss and vitality, only to find that after a few weeks or months of cutting calories to a ridiculous low, exercising like crazy, counting every gram and morsel that entered your mouth, and constantly obsessing about making the right choice, you stepped on the scale and saw only the slightest weight loss? And how many times have you noticed that all that great vitality you thought you'd be feeling as a result of your new diet never shows up, that instead you're left feeling exhausted, cranky, and always starving?

If you're like most people, this isn't an unfamiliar experience at all. In fact, it's so common that it's the reason people no longer believe in diets. Well, I don't blame them. The fact is, a diet will never solve your weight loss and health problems, simply because almost every kind of diet out there demands that you eat, live, work out, and plan your every bite in a completely unnatural, unsustainable way.

The 16/8 method of intermittent fasting is the exact opposite of dieting. It doesn't force you to change everything you eat, count a single calorie or obsess about how much exercise you need to be doing to meet your goal. Instead, the most basic version of 16/8 simply requires that you make one small change: your eating schedule.

The 16/8 in the plan's name stands for the fact that on it, you'll be fasting for 16 hours a day and feeding for 8 hours a day. Now, I know what you're thinking: 16 entire hours of fasting doesn't sound like just one small change! I'll bet you're thinking it actually sounds worse than any diet out there but trust me, it's one of the simplest, most intuitive moves you can make and it's far easier to pull off than you can imagine.

That's because, although 16 hours sounds like a lot, you'll actually be asleep for at least 8 out of the 16 fasting hours. The so-called"16 hour" fast actually begins after your last meal at night at 8 or 9 PM and ends at 12 noon or 1 pm the next day when you have lunch as the first meal of your day. We'll get into the real nitty-gritty of how to successfully pull off the 16/8 fast a little later in this chapter, but first, I want to fill you in on WHY 16/8 is such an effective method of weight loss, and why it's my favorite type of intermittent fast for longevity, energy, mental clarity, and a whole host of other bonuses.

How Does 16/8 Work?

The easiest way to answer this question would be to say, it works intuitively. Why? Simply because this is how our bodies used to function, before the availability of endless amounts of food made us into all-day feeders. As I explained in previous sections, we were once hunter-gatherers who set off early in the day without breakfast. We would then seek food for several hours and by the time we'd finished finding it, preparing it, and eating it, it would already be well past mid-day. Because our ancestors never ate late into the evening as we mindlessly do now, their last meal of the previous day would certainly have been no later than 8 PM. That means after hunting and gathering all morning the next day, when they finally did eat, they would have already spent at least 16 hours fasting. "Well, so what?" you might ask. "That doesn't necessarily mean that the old way is the right way." In this case, as in so many other cases, the old way is indeed not only the right way, but the only way.

You see, two things have changed drastically since the days of hunting and gathering. Mankind has never been so sick and overweight before, and mankind has also never been so abundantly overfed before. Trust me, this is no coincidence. These two facts are certainly intertwined. Today we're told to always be prepared to eat by having up to 6 entire meals in one day! We're told that our bodies need this type of frequent eating to survive. But do you think our ancestors were lugging around coolers and baggies of prepped snacks with them in the wilderness? We don't even have to go that far back. Do you think our great-grandparents' generation ran around taking breaks to eat their 6 supposedly "necessary" meals a day? The answer is: absolutely not. And yet, neither our ancient ancestors nor our great-grandparents were overweight or plagued by the chronic inflammatory diseases we suffer from today. You'll find from historical writings that many people in the past didn't consume breakfast and instead ate lunch and an early dinner. Did they die?

Were they unable to think clearly, live fully, or achieve? No, in fact, there's reason to believe that eating less frequently actually helped them to function better mentally, physically, and even emotionally. Let's look at the difference between grazing all day and eating only intermittently.

Burning Fat: Fat is the best possible fuel for our bodies to burn. When you burn fat, you're getting a calm, steady source of energy that provides you with vitality and strength for hours on end. On the hand, when you burn sugar, you're getting a quick, explosion of frantic energy that burns out super-fast, leaving you more tired and sick than ever before.

Burning sugar leads to a buildup of deadly toxins and a backlog of dangerous diseases, but burning fat is actually deeply purifying and removes built-up acids and other undesirable substances. So now that we've established fat as the clear winner in the best fuel contest, let's talk about why our ancestors were able to burn fat and why we aren't able to do so as efficiently. To put it bluntly, eating all day has caused us to lose our ability to burn fat for energy. Instead, we just store fat away and burn sugar instead, leading to ballooning weight and a plethora of health problems. When the body receives food every couple of hours, it has no need to dig deep and burn its fat stores for energy. Instead it burns the easily available fuel from the food it keeps getting fed. Usually, because it gets quite a lot of food so often and doesn't do the kind of tough physical work that our ancestors did, the body will then store any excess energy from the food into itself as—you guessed it—FAT. Now, we have a situation where not only is the body no longer burning its already large stores of fat for energy, but by being frequently fed, it's actually adding to those stores of fat! The New York Academy of Sciences even published a report showing that eating all-day led to an increased risk of heart disease, stroke, and type 2 diabetes.

And this is not just conjecture. The facts are there for anyone who cares to look. Studies show that when people reduced the number of meals they ate a day (even if they ate the same amount of total calories) for just two weeks, they lost a significant amount of weight, improved their energy levels, their cognitive abilities, their moods, and were able to cut down their cravings! Why did this happen? Because they were going for longer in between meals, their body switched from burning the easy cheap sugar energy from constant meals to burning their own fat stores. Suddenly, even without adding exercise or cutting the number of calories they consumed in a day, these people were losing weight and drastically improving their health, with just one simple change.

That's what 16/8 is all about—one shift that will then totally revolutionize the way you look, feel and live. When you fast for 16 hours between dinner and lunch, your body is freed up from digesting and metabolizing, and can turn its attention to repairing and rebooting. Evidence shows us that those who fast intermittently by eating fewer meals gain a myriad of benefits including:

- Reduced inflammation
- Reduced blood pressure and cholesterol levels
- Metabolism enhanced by entering ketosis, or optimal fat-burning state
- Significant weight loss that is easy to maintain
- Prevention of, improvement in and even total elimination of type 2 diabetes
- Lower blood sugar levels and enhanced insulin sensitivity
- Strengthened heart
- Elimination of deadly visceral fat
- Increased memory and learning ability
- Decreased depression and anxiety

I recommend 16/8 fasting because it is effective while also being satiating and making it easy for you to continue to work and play as usual. But all types of intermittent fasts reduce oxidative stress by lowering the accumulation of oxidative radicals in your cells.

This helps to prevent oxidative damage from happening to your cells' proteins, nucleic acids, and lipids. Because oxidative stress and damage play a huge role in causing us to age and to become ill, fasting intermittently is a powerful way to stem the tide of premature aging and disease. In addition to this, every time you fast, you are inducing a mild and beneficial cellular stress response that helps your cells to fend off illnesses and rapid aging in the same way that exercise does. By the way, I highly recommend adding some exercise to any fasting protocol you use in order to get a double whammy of benefits. I'll talk more about this later in the book, so stay tuned.

So now that you're fully informed and revved up to try your hand at 16/8 fasting, let's get into the best way to do so.

A typical day on the 16/8 fast goes like this:

You wake up and instead of making a meal, you have a cup of coffee, tea, or any other non-caloric beverage. Then around 12 noon, you sit down to a large meal. From this point on, you're free to eat as usual until 8 PM, when you should have had your last meal of the day. You head off to bed and sleep for 8 hours and obviously during this period, you aren't eating anything.

When you wake up in the morning, simply by pushing your first meal of the day back until 12 noon, you've just completed a 16 hour fast. Your feeding period is an 8 hour window in which you can eat freely without counting a single calorie or worrying about fitting in a certain amount of exercise. You don't starve yourself, you don't measure your meals, and yet, you lose more weight than you ever could on even the lowest calorie diet.

It's as easy as that, and as a major fan of this form of IF myself, I can tell you that not only have I seen amazing results in others who've tried the 16/8 method, I've never seen any other way of eating that allows you to lose up to 4 pounds in less than a week, without the usual torture that comes with dieting!

And the beauty of the 16/8 fasting method is that you get to choose how many times you'd like to do it within a week. Some people start off by fasting in this way for only a couple days a week while some do it every other day of the week and with its ease, many people prefer to eat in the 16/8 way every day. The best part is that whichever schedule you choose, 16/8 is one of the most effective IF methods and people see real results much faster than they ever expected. However, my personal recommendation is that even if you have to do it gradually, you should work towards making the 16/8 schedule your every day meal plan.

That's because the more often you limit your eating time to an 8 hour period, the sooner you start to see amazing benefits, from pounds that practically fly off you, to plunging blood sugar, better mental clarity and concentration, and even an improved mood.

Debunking the Breakfast Myth

Now I can almost hear the horrified nutritionists out there gasping: "But what about breakfast, the most important meal of the day?" Well, I'm going to let you in on one secret that could mean the difference between being overweight, unhealthy, and tired, or lean, fit, and full of energy: DON'T EAT BREAKFAST!

Let me start out by debunking the tired old myth that we've all been taught: ignore what you read on the back of your cereal box. Breakfast is NOT some essential meal that human beings simply can't live without. In fact, historically and biologically, we don't do well on breakfast at all because it doesn't work with our physiological makeup. Our bodies actually reject eating in the morning. Don't believe it? Think about this:

Haven't you ever had the kind of good solid breakfast that many nutritionists recommend and then found yourself absolutely starving after only an hour or two? Don't you notice that on days when you're running late and have to miss your morning meal, you find yourself less hungry and weirdly less tired than usual?

Well, it's not just your imagination and you're certainly not alone. Breakfast triggers our appetites and can keep us in a hungry, fatigued state for the rest of the day!

Here's why: While we've always been told that having a square morning meal is the best way to get our day started off properly, the truth is it's a recipe for illness, weight gain, and fatigue. When we eat first thing in the AM, we are essentially working against our body's natural processes. The morning is when our circadian cortisol cycle hits its highest point, meaning that this is when our levels of the stress hormone cortisol are at their peak.

This may not seem like a particularly big problem until you realize that this high cortisol point causes our bodies to release way too much insulin when we scarf down any type of breakfast, even if it's a super healthy meal. When this rush of insulin is released, blood glucose levels plunge suddenly, causing exhaustion, a cranky and less than stable mood and, you guessed it—a massive hunger attack. This doesn't occur in the same way during any other time of the day, so clearly a morning meal first thing is not going to help us keep our blood sugar levels steady and our hunger at bay, as we've been wrongly told so often by the experts.

Research is now finally catching up to what so many people have been claiming for years. One recent study pointed out that those who didn't eat breakfast tended to consume fewer calories during the day than those who started off their days with a morning meal. Other studies have shown that those who use the 16/8 method to skip breakfast show a dramatic improvement in cholesterol levels, inflammation markers, and also lose more weight than they would by simply restricting calories. *This is huge: you can lose more weight by passing up breakfast than by dieting all day, even if you actually eat more food than you would if you were dieting!* This just goes to prove that insulin control is one of the most important benefits of the 16/8 intermittent fast method.

With the popularity of intermittent fasting on the rise, new results are coming in all the time. So far, tests show us that missing breakfast can:

- Decrease hunger, limit cravings and lower the amount of food you eat
- Rev up fat breakdown
- Improve insulin and blood glucose stability
- Stimulate the secretion of human growth hormone (HGH), leading to weight loss and better health
- Protect your heart from disease

From a personal point of view, after many years of following conventional guidelines and never missing my breakfast, I began to see that both the scientific research and my own as well as others' experiences were showing that this was majorly unhealthy.

I now no longer eat breakfast unless I'm pulling a particularly strenuous workload and know that I won't be able to fit in a meal unless I do. It was hard at first to get rid of the misconception that missing breakfast was supposedly the most damaging things a person could do to their body and health, but after just a few breakfast-free days, I felt light, energetic and most importantly, I didn't find myself craving more food all day long. From then on, I knew that I wouldn't be going back to force-feeding my body an early morning meal it didn't even want or need. I know this is going to be a tough step for a lot of people because, after all, we've all been raised on the belief that breakfast is somehow more important than any other meal. If you have a hard time just axing your morning meal right off the bat, I suggest that you try to roll it back gradually, by eating smaller portions or pushing back your normal breakfast time by a few hours.

But I will say this: if you bravely take the plunge and miss a couple of days of breakfast, you will see immediate results. You'll feel less hungry, you'll be bursting with vitality, and you may even notice some weight loss in the first few days. That's because, with breakfast out of the way, your body will no longer be releasing huge amounts of insulin to cope with that unnecessary early morning meal. Once you see the amazing benefits of not forcing breakfast on your body when it doesn't need it, you'll never look back!

I know that many people have a hard time getting the energy they need to get their day started and many people view breakfast as a way to fuel themselves through the morning. But the truth is that when you "fuel" yourself with a carb-rich, starchy or heavy meal in the morning, you're really only spiking your blood sugar and giving yourself an unnatural and short lived sense of energy. After less than half an hour, your body's natural circadian cortisol response will flush you with an overdose of insulin that will send your blood sugar plunging and your energy levels will be far worse than before you ate.

Still, going breakfast free doesn't mean that you have to go fuel–free. I'm going to share with you one of the biggest IF hacks out there that will totally revolutionize the way you see your mornings and the way you think, concentrate and feel in the early hours. And it's super delicious, too!

Ready? The secret is coffee, and not just any old coffee—IF, fat burning, metabolism boosting, concentration enhancing, energy-giving coffee! This coffee is so effective, so filling, and so absolutely tasty that most people who replace their normal breakfast with it regret that they didn't know about it sooner.

So what's in this special coffee? To be honest, it's a very simple, pure recipe. It's not some mass produced "health" supplement drink that you have to go out and buy. Chances are you have everything you need to make this awesome cup of joe in your kitchen right now. All you need is some good quality butter (preferably grass-fed), coconut oil, and coffee. Seriously, that's it!

So what makes this the best way to replace breakfast? Well, for starters, grass-fed butter is chock full of the perfect fats our bodies need to fight off bad cholesterol and a great omega-3 to omega-6 fatty acid balance, which makes it absolutely fantastic at gearing the body up to reduce body fat. And if that wasn't enough, the combination of CLA and ketone-producing healthy fats in the butter and coconut oil are intense inflammation-fighters that have been proven to cut down body fat mass, particularly in those who are overweight.

What about energy? Well, there's a reason this coffee brew is replacing energy drinks for thousands of fitness and health-minded people (and practically all the tech geniuses out in Silicon Valley, too!). It's loaded with beneficial short-chain fatty acids that increase energy levels and give you plenty of mental clarity and focus for up to 6 hours after just one cup! (If you want to give this coffee mix a try as a replacement for your usual big breakfast, I've added my special recipe for it in the recipe index you'll find at the end of this book. Just remember not to have more than one very small cup during your fasting periods, as it does contain a higher calorie count. Still, if you find yourself too hungry or too tired to focus when you first start 16/8 fasting, this coffee makes for a great way to ease your body into the transition of not eating breakfast!)

Never Break Your Fast With Carbohydrates!

Now that we've got breakfast out of the way, let me say a few words about what I recommend regarding your other meals. When it comes to food choices on the 16/8 version of intermittent fasting, the reason we say it's not a diet is because it really is up to you what you eat during your 8 hour feeding window. Unlike other plans, you won't be measuring, counting and obsessing about macros. Still, with that said, I do want to let you in on my top tip for the best possible results on the 16/8 plan—kick carbs out. I don't mean that you shouldn't have any carbohydrates at all. I just mean that when it comes to breaking your fast with your first meal of the day, you should definitely grab something loaded with protein and healthy fats, like a nice juicy steak and some free-range eggs, along with a portion of low GI vegetables such as asparagus spears or a spinach salad, instead of a carbohydrate-packed option like bread or white rice. This is because carbs, as I'll mention many times in this book, actually have the power to reverse a lot of the best benefits of your intermittent fast. One of the main reasons that the 16/8 intermittent fasting method works is because it powerfully controls your insulin levels. Whenever you eat a high carbohydrate meal, you're basically cancelling out this wonderful benefit. Insulin is a fat storing hormone, and the moment your body starts taking in and metabolizing carbs, it begins to overproduce insulin. The simplest way to understand this is with this formula: more carbs lead to more insulin, and more insulin leads to more weight gain, more hunger pangs, high blood pressure, rapid aging, and a shortened lifespan.

These effects are exactly what intermittent fasting corrects, so in order to truly get the best benefits out of your fast, I recommend that you never break a fast with a high-carbohydrate meal, and that you generally follow a low-carb, high fat menu during your feeding hours.

Now, in the interest of full disclosure, I do want you to know that there are plenty of people who go on a 16/8 fast and scarf down a box of donuts during their feeding period. A lot of them actually still lose weight because IF is just so effective, but they don't lose as much as they should be losing and they certainly don't get all of the brain boosting, longevity-promoting and anti-aging effects they should be getting. I want you to get the full benefits of your fast, not just a couple of pounds here and there and I want you to feel, function, and look great while you're doing it.

Because studies show us that a low-carb way of eating leaves you with lower insulin levels both when you're fasting and when you're feeding, this is the best possible way to really get the fat loss, energy, health and longevity you're looking for.

Does This Mean Absolutely No Carbs?

Not at all. There are plenty of good carbohydrates that I urge you to include in your meal plans. While bad carbs spike your blood sugar and cause massive insulin releases, good carbs don't raise blood sugar as high or as rapidly. The very best carbs you can add to your meals are non-starchy vegetables. These are loaded with highly nourishing vitamins, minerals and phytochemicals—plant compounds that keep you safe from inflammation, cardiovascular diseases, rapid aging, and even cancer. They also provide a great supply of fiber to ensure that everything moves along well. This is particularly important when doing intermittent fasting because the lack of constant feeding can, at first, leave people a little irregular. The fiber in veggies will correct that for you quickly and naturally.

To make your choice easier for you, I've created this list of excellent carbohydrates to include during the feeding portion of your intermittent fasts:

- Artichokes
- Asparagus
- Broccoli
- Brussels sprouts
- Cabbage (all varieties are great)
- Cauliflower
- Celery
- Cucumber
- Eggplant
- Leeks
- Lentils
- Beans (kidney, garbanzo and green beans, in particular)

- Greens (this includes mustard greens, kale and collard greens)
- Mushrooms
- Okra
- Onions
- Peppers
- Radishes
- Spinach
- Squash
- Swiss chard
- Tomato
- Watercress and all other salad greens (including romaine, iceberg lettuce, chicory and arugula)
- Zucchini

When it comes to fruit, your best choices are:

- Apples and pears
- Apricots

- Berries (including raspberries, blueberries, strawberries, black berries, gooseberries, huckleberries)
- Cherries
- Grapefruit
- Peaches
- Figs

<u>My Top Tips For A Successful 16/8 Fast:</u>

<u>Tip# 1: Find The Timing That Works Best For You, But Stick As Closely To An 8 Hour Feeding Window As Possible</u> The example I give here is based on my own 16/8 fasting schedule, but that doesn't mean that you have to eat dinner at 8 PM the night before and break your fast at 12 noon. That's just how I do it, but you can choose to eat dinner at, say, 9 PM the night before and break your fast the next day at 1 PM, or you can eat dinner at 7:45 PM and break your fast at 11:45 AM the next day. Some people even extend their fast from 16 hours to 18 or even 20 hours. They do so by eating dinner the previous night at 8 PM and then not eating anything until 18 or 20 hours later, the next day.

This is an extreme method that really only works for a small handful of people and not one I personally recommend, as it doesn't allow the 8 hour window of feeding which research shows us is part of the reason the 16/8 fast works so well. But it really is up to you, how your body feels, and your particular schedule. And of course, fasting on a slightly modified plan is way more beneficial than not fasting at all because you couldn't fit it in to your day!

Tip # 2: Breakup With Breakfast For Good The one caveat is that whichever schedule you choose for yourself, you'll need to still avoid eating breakfast (or any morning meal that takes place a couple of hours after you've woken up) for the cortisol and insulin reasons I explained previously AND you'll also want to avoid eating anything in the three hours before you go to sleep.

<u>Tip # 3: For Faster Weight Loss, Better Anti-inflammatory Effects and Enhanced Brain Function and Mood, Aim For High Protein, High Fat and Low Carb Meals</u>

As you know by now, intermittent fasting on the 16/8 plan is so effective that you could be gorging on a carb-fest during your feeding periods and you'd probably still see pretty great weight loss results, due to the way this fast forces your body to switch from burning glucose to burning your own stores of body fat. But, and this is a big but, you wouldn't be making the most of all the health benefits provided by intermittent fasting if you were to eat like that. That's because a large amount of carbohydrates, particularly simple carbs, causes spikes in your blood sugar, triggers insulin rushes, and switches on your inflammatory responses. Now, intermittent fasting has been shown to work very effectively to cool inflammation, but if you're constantly switching on the inflammation that the fast is trying to switch off, eventually, inflammation will win out. No matter how healing this fasting method is, if you repeatedly allow yourself to eat too much of the foods that cause illness, all the intermittent fasting in the world won't be of much use.

That's why I strongly recommend that those who want to lose a larger amount of weight, those who have chronic illnesses of any kind and type 2 diabetes in particular, and those who really need to see an improvement in brain function, mix this fast method with a generally low carb meal plan. You should be getting the majority of your carbohydrate intake from low GI, non-starchy vegetables and a limited portion of fruits. Other than that, feel free to eat as much delicious fat and protein as your heart desires. If you're worried about going hungry during feeding periods, remember that eating low carb, high fat meals is actually much more satisfying than eating high carb, low fat meals. Think about it—when you're absolutely ravenous what would you rather have, a dry bagel or bacon, extra helpings of butter, and a steak as large as you like?

Tip # 4: If You're Eating Low Carb, Don't Stress About Calories Or Portion Control

This tip is linked to the one above. While the vast majority of people on the 16/8 fast do remarkably well and stick with it, the few cases I've seen where that hasn't happened have been because of one thing and one thing alone: counting calories and cutting portions.

Simply put, if you turn this fasting method into just another low calorie diet where you have to run around measuring, counting, and worrying about everything you put in your mouth, it will end up failing, just like any low calorie diet. The reason so many people stick with intermittent fasting on the 16/8 method and see results that last is because it is NOT a diet. You'll be far more likely to last through your 16 hour fast period if you know that you have a satisfying amount of food waiting for you during your 8 hour feeding period. Your body will also understand that it is being nourished and taken care of and won't try to hold on to any fat unnecessarily. If, on the other hand, you start trying to cut calories drastically and limit portions, two things will happen: 1: Your body will start to suffer from the strain of fasting AND being on a low calorie diet, which is a combo I never recommend. 2: Your will-power and enthusiasm will take a hit from all the usual things that make dieting impossible to succeed at, such as counting, measuring, and worrying. The trick with IF is that it feels intuitive. When your fast is up, you eat real, whole, and wholly satisfying meals until you are totally satiated.

Your body was made to fast and feast cyclically, and it truly responds well to this type of meal plan. Don't let years of dieting hype get into your head and confuse you. Listen to your body and you'll see those pounds slipping away while you remain nourished, fed, energetic, and healthy!

Join me in the next chapter for an eye-opening look at how intermittent fasting can literally wipe out one of the biggest killers of our time!

Chapter 7: Intermittent Fasting—Kiss Diabetes and Blood Glucose Disorders Goodbye!

One of the biggest lies we've been fed in recent years is that our brains can't function without glucose as its fuel. This has led to many people desperately trying to "keep up" their blood sugar levels by snacking throughout the day. Even when they are eating so called healthy snacks, they are still doing irreparable harm to their bodies, their minds, and their long term longevity.

One of the most important things I want to take away from this chapter is this message—the human brain DOES NOT need a big supply of glucose in order to operate. In fact, glucose is like cheap, unfiltered fuel. It may be easily available but it should never be your first choice for energy. Unfortunately, decades of nutritionists recommending diets that include regular supposedly "healthy" mini-meals made up of carb-loaded, sugar-rich foods like granola, dried fruit, and other glucose traps have left people munching all day and every bite is taking us one step closer to one of the biggest killers of our time—diabetes!

Let me give you an example of this misguided information: have you ever told your doctor that you wanted to go on a completely sugar-free diet or even searched conventional health websites about this type of diet? I'm almost certain that you've been warned against going too far with eating sugar-free with a line that goes something like, "Glucose is your brain's primary fuel and is important for proper functioning—as long as you don't go overboard, sugar can play a healthy role in your diet." This is the same kind of excuse that people often give when they tell you why they can't go on an intermittent fast. You see, for so long we've believed that keeping our brains and bodies fuelled with glucose through near continuous snacking and the outdated idea of "three solid meals" is absolutely necessary,

It's time to debunk this dangerous concept here and now—glucose is not the elite wonder fuel that lazy science has made it out to be for so many years, and when you fast, you are not putting your body and mind at risk. Quite the contrary is true.

Now, we know that the brain generally does well on about 30 grams of glucose on very high fat, low-carb diets, such as those eating a traditional Inuit diet or going on extreme Paleo. So where does this glucose come from? Not from sugary foods, not from starchy carbs, but from your own body! When your body enters a deeply fasted state it can actually make up to 21% of its own glucose supply by burning fat. When you fast, your body produces glycerol, which supplies a lot of the glucose your brain uses for energy. The rest can easily be made up from your regular diet and does not require you to go on some crazy nutritionist-approved all day carb fest.

So the next time someone tells you that going on an intermittent fasting plan is dangerous because it will eliminate your body's glucose supply, tell them that your own body is very capable of fulfilling the small need for glucose it has and that you don't need to be eating all day, every day, non-stop, to be healthy. A simple look at the way our ancestors lived is more than enough to illustrate this point. How many hunter-gatherers do you think were walking around in the forest snacking on glucose-packed food all day and stopping their activities to eat three square meals? The answer is almost certainly none, and if our ancestors didn't need to worry about skipping a meal or two, we definitely are capable of doing the same without any harmful side effects. One major difference between the way we live now and the way we used to live is that, back in those days, a disease like diabetes simply couldn't have taken hold and spread like it's doing today. And the reason is this— we ate for nutrition, when our bodies needed it, and NOT by some arbitrary schedule that forces us to keep ourselves in a fed state for far too much of the time.

This continuous feeding has left us with a massive diabetes problem on our hands. 371 million people globally now have this terrifying condition and that number looks set to multiply rapidly. In just the last 10 years, the rate of new diabetes cases has risen 90%! And all the evidence points to one truth we can't ignore: if we keep doing what we've been doing, we'll keep seeing epidemic levels of diabetes! That's really why intermittent fasting is so important. Not only is it the complete opposite of all the stale medical advice we now know doesn't work, it has also been proven to wipe out diabetes.

Now, fasting as a cure for diabetes is not a new concept. Historically, fasting has always been seen as the best medicine for illness of almost every kind, and all the way back in 1906, the famed world-leading diabetes expert Dr. Elliot Joslin posited that fasting was the perfect cure for diabetes. Somehow, this knowledge was lost along the way and since then, we've been effectively feeding the monster that is diabetes. So how does intermittent fasting work? It starves type 2 diabetes right into nonexistence by removing its true root causes, chronic inflammation and insulin resistance.

Now, this is the complete opposite of the accepted advice from most doctors and nutritionists. They tell us that diabetics need to be eating frequently and regularly throughout the day in order to stabilize their blood sugar levels and combat insulin resistance. But if that was true, the millions of people who have been carefully following this misguided diet would have seen improvements in their diabetes. Instead, their insulin resistance has only gotten worse, their blood sugar is impossible to control, they're putting on pounds, and they've been told that their situation is incurable–that it will just go on and on and perhaps end up being the cause of an early death.

Well, if this sounds terrifyingly familiar, I'd like to tell you that this is not true at all. Your condition is <u>definitely controllable</u> and <u>even reversible,</u> once you let go of the commonly prescribed myths about the right way to eat for diabetes. Intermittent fasting has provided many people with supposedly "uncontrollable" diabetes with a fast, effective solution that works without medication. Still, conventional medicine insists that fasting is not the answer for stable blood sugar and that in fact, it could even be dangerous to diabetics!

But the evidence tells us a totally different story: a number of studies have shown that far from being a cause of high blood sugar and insulin issues, intermittent fasting actually lowers blood sugar long term, and completely eliminates insulin resistance! In a recent study, those with type 2 diabetes tried intermittent fasting for three days and immediately displayed much lower blood glucose levels as well as increased insulin sensitivity. In another test, type 2 diabetics who went beyond the normal 12 hour period of not eating overnight, by not eating for 18 hours, showed an astonishing 23% drop in blood glucose! Those who engaged in a once a week 24 hour fast displayed a sharp fall in levels of blood glucose and up to a 31 % drop in insulin levels!

Intermittent Fasting and Weight Loss:

As we know, weight loss is a major goal for most people with type 2 diabetes. That's because any extra weight can actually spike insulin resistance, making it impossible for the body to use insulin correctly. Intermittent fasting does wonders in this area too. After just a short period of fasting intermittently, your body's levels of human growth hormone (HGH) shoot up as much as 5-fold. This is extremely beneficial for weight loss, because HGH promotes the burning of fat, resulting in rapid weight loss. Intermittent fasting brings down insulin levels while simultaneously increasing amounts of the hormone norepinephrine, and both of these actions help your body metabolize fat and use it as an energy source.

In addition to this, tests show that short bouts of intermittent fasting can actually raise your metabolism by almost 4%, making calorie-burning and weight loss extremely easy.

Another way that IF combats diabetes through weight loss is by causing targeted weight loss in the abdominal area. Those fasting intermittently showed an average 4 to 7% loss in waist size. Research has long pointed to abdominal fat as a culprit in the development and worsening of type 2 diabetes, so by busting belly fat, IF is also eliminating the conditions that cause diabetes.

And the best part is that these results are consistent across the board, whether you choose a 24 hour fast, an alternate day fast, or any of the other fasting methods.

So what does this tell us? No matter which type of intermittent fasting method you choose, all provide viable treatment options for type 2 diabetes that work far better than the common treatments on the market now.

Still, even with all of these amazing rewards, there are some risks to consider when it comes to starting any new eating plan with diabetes. With that in mind, I've laid out a detailed plan to help you fast intermittently with greater success and safety.

Fasting With Diabetes:

What's The Best Type Of Intermittent Fast for Me, As A Type 2 Diabetic?

While all types of IF are incredibly healthful and have shown both in real life case studies and in scientific research to have an excellent effect on those with type 2 diabetes, I do have a personal favorite when it comes to lowering insulin resistance and speeding up weight loss while making it easy to stay on track. This is the 16/8 type of fast, in which you simply limit the hours in the day in which you can eat. Please head to the earlier chapters in this book where I go in-depth about how to get the best results out of this type of fast for more information.

Important Note: It's absolutely critical to keep in mind that intermittent fasting is a great treatment option for type 2 diabetes but that it is **NOT** normally recommended for those with type 1 diabetes.

If you attempt to try IF with type 1 diabetes, there's a serious risk that your blood glucose levels may shoot up too high and lead to hyperglycemia. This in turn will cause substances called ketones to build up in your system, leading to a dangerous condition called diabetic ketoacidosis.

If you are currently using insulin to control your type 2 diabetes, it's a good idea to speak with your doctor before you begin your fast, as sudden changes in your eating can affect insulin levels dramatically— meaning that intermittent fasting may make you suddenly too healthy for the amount of medication you're taking.

The Secret to Successfully Fasting With Type 2 Diabetes:

Follow these top tips to make sure that your intermittent fasting kicks type 2 diabetes out of your life for good!

Take It Slow In the Beginning:

While IF is definitely a highly effective treatment, type 2 diabetes is still a tricky and serious condition, and it's important to understand that the levels of insulin already in your body may make it difficult for you to get into fat-burning mode right away. This doesn't mean that you won't get the results you want. It only means that you may need to start slowly. One great way of doing this is to cut down the fasting periods a little, allowing your body to ease into the process.

Cut Back on Carbohydrates:

This is something I advise everyone starting intermittent fasting to do, but it's all the more essential for those with type 2 diabetes. While you've probably heard that complex carbs are an essential part of a healthy diet for those with diabetes, this just isn't true. No matter how complex the carb you're eating, it can still place a lot of strain on your maxed out body by creating a need for more and more insulin, leaving you ill, fatigued, overweight, and burned out.

In order to make sure your blood glucose levels don't spiral out of hand, you should begin all intermittent fasting with a brief period of low to no-carbohydrate meals. This also applies to days when you're fasting, as well as those when you aren't, because cutting carbs is the key to keeping your glucose in check while also entering a slightly ketogenic state and facilitating weight loss. If you don't do this, you'll find yourself struggling to enter the fat burning phase, while also placing your health in danger with the possibility of high blood sugar levels.

When cutting carbs, try to keep your total carb intake well below the 100 grams a day line, and always select foods with low glycemic loads and indexes.

Try Out Various Types of Intermittent Fasting and Choose the Right One for You:

As you know, IF isn't a one-size-fits-all process. There are different ways to fast intermittently and each method has its benefits and potential drawbacks, depending on your unique makeup and condition. Reactions to fasting differ widely among people, so it's crucial to really notice how you feel with each type of fast and make a selection based on how your body responds. I recommend that you begin with an IF fast that allows you to eat a limited amount of calories a day, rather than a full, no calorie fast. This will ensure that your blood glucose levels remain steady throughout.

Exercise While You Fast for the Best Results:

Boost your type 2 diabetes-busting results by adding a little exercise to the mix. Working out while you're still fasting takes blood sugar lowering and insulin sensitivity to a whole new level, making sure you get the very best out of your IF efforts.

Because your blood sugar levels tend to be higher in the mornings, it's a great idea to exercise first thing in the morning on an empty stomach for maximum fat burning and blood sugar decreasing effects.

Never Break Your Fast with a High-Carb Meal

All people on an intermittent fast should aim to steer clear of carbs when breaking their fasts, but when it comes to those with type 2 diabetes, breaking a fast with high-carb foods can spell major disaster. I cannot stress this enough—not only should you be combining your IF with a low-carb eating plan, you should NEVER reach for a carb as your first post-fast meal. This is because carbohydrates are essentially sugar in chain form, so as you eat them, they immediately spike your blood glucose and make your insulin resistance much worse.

Whichever IF schedule you follow, remember that your blood glucose levels will often be highest in the morning as your liver is busy making sugar overnight. Due to this, I recommend that your initial meal should be protein and fat-loaded and as low in carb content as possible, in order to switch off your liver's sugar production. A great way to you break your fast is with a handful of nuts, or go for eggs, meats, and other rich sources of protein, while avoiding foods that are high GI. After your initial meal of the day, you should be able to supplement your intake with small portions of non-starchy, low GI vegetables and fruits.

Keep An Eye On Your Medication Levels:

This is something I mentioned briefly above but it's so important that I want to touch on it again. When it comes to type 2 diabetes, intermittent fasting works—I mean, *really* works. Even from your first fast day, you'll likely see your blood glucose drop much lower than you've seen them go before. This means that on fast days, you may need to adjust your doses of medication because IF is so effective at doing what your meds are trying to do that adding both fasting and medication together may result in dangerously low blood glucose levels. In fact, I know of one woman who had been a type 2 diabetic for over 30 years and always had stubbornly high blood glucose levels. When someone introduced her to intermittent fasting, she was shocked by the results she saw!

Her usually sky-high blood glucose levels had dropped so low that she couldn't believe what she was seeing. She consulted with her doctor and he told her that IF was doing such a great job of lowering her blood glucose levels that he was going to have to lower the amount of medication she was taking for her diabetes—because IF and the medication together would have been too much. She continued with fasting intermittently and within months was able to gradually decrease and then eliminate her medication altogether.

This is just one case but I've experienced so many are just like it that I'm confident you'll begin to see quite a huge change in your blood glucose levels very early on. Monitor yourself closely and talk with your doctor to make sure reducing your dosage is the best move for you.

The only case where I don't believe any medication dosage changes are required is when it comes to metformin. Metformin is a medication that works to reduce insulin resistance and can be a great part of your health plan, side by side with IF and eating low-carb. When your insulin resistance fades away through continued intermittent fasting, you'll likely get the go ahead from your doctor to adjust or eliminate Metformin too, but again, it's absolutely crucial that you talk to you doctor before making any changes on your own.

Watch Out for Hypoglycemia:

Some of the medications you may be taking for your diabetes could end up causing episodes of extremely low blood sugar, otherwise known as hypoglycemia. The medications most likely to do this are sulphonylureas such as glyclopyramide, glibenclamide, glyburide, glibornuride, gliclazide, glipizide, glibornuride, gliquidone, glisoxepide, and glimepiride. Because IF causes your insulin resistance to be lowered as you fast, these medications may cause your pancreas to release more insulin than you actually need.

If your blood sugar levels drop drastically, you may need to take in some carbs in the short term. In the long term, you will need to speak with your doctor about reducing your medication dosages, so that you can continue to fast intermittently and remain on a low-carb eating plan, in order to completely control and reverse your type 2 diabetes!

If this is the beginning of your IF journey to healing your type 2 diabetes, then I am very excited for you. You'll be seeing changes and improvements in your health, body, appearance, mood, and mind that many doctors falsely told you were nearly impossible. Remember to keep monitoring your blood glucose and to add in exercise and you'll really be on your way to a diabetes-free future, in a truly safe, natural, and effective way!

So intermittent fasting works wonders for your body, but what about your brain? Make sure to check out the following chapter to find out all about its brain-saving benefits!

Chapter 8: The Brain Boost—How Intermittent Fasting Can Help You Improve Your Memory, Think More Clearly, and Protect Your Brain From Disease And Depression

If I asked you to name some of your biggest health fears surrounding aging, I'm willing to bet that dementia, memory loss, or any other cognitive disorders would definitely be in the top ten. Why? Well, quite simply, cognitive disorders have reached an all-time high. We've come to accept that everyone will eventually end up losing their mental faculties, becoming dependent on others to carry out even the most basic tasks and being incapable of caring for themselves. As you read this, nearly 50 million people suffer from dementia worldwide and there are over 7 million new cases every year! While plenty of people are turning to intermittent fasting, looking for a solution to weight gain, fatigue, and other concerns, a growing number are also seeking it out in order to literally rescue their brains!

You've probably heard all of the hype about the right way to tune up your brain and protect yourself from age-related cognitive decline, right? "Eat plenty of fish, eat fat, don't eat fat, gorge on kale, stuff yourself on eggs, go vegan, go Paleo!"

When it comes to brain health, it seems like every new piece of advice you hear from doctors, nutritionists, and diet specialists seems to directly contradict previous recommendations, making it easy to be confused and left wondering if nutrition really has anything to do with a healthy mind at all. Well, I've got a very clear, short, and simple answer for you. It's really *how* and *when* you eat that matters most to your brain, rather than *what* you eat. If you want to boost your brain cells, stay mentally young, and keep a whole slew of dangerous brain-draining diseases such as Alzheimer's, depression, and even various types of psychiatric disorders at bay, forget about chasing down the latest super food or diet. Instead, focus on harnessing the power of one of the most ancient and simple healing tools that mankind has—fasting.

I know, it sounds pretty tough to believe. After all, we've all spent decades hearing that this meal plan or that particular ingredient is the key to healing our brains. Recently however, study after scientific study has come out proving that in fact, the LESS frequently you feed the brain, the better it functions. Now, I'm not saying that you should try starving yourself in order to smarten up or keep your wits sharp. That would actually be counter-productive because our brains require a certain level of caloric intake to fuel their functions and keep them in top condition. Additionally, our brains are largely made up of fatty tissues and would likely shrivel up from a very low-calorie or low-fat diet.

What I *am* saying, and what doctors, nutritionists, and scientists around the world have begun to espouse, is that fasting intermittently is the ideal way to help your brain work at maximum speed, efficiency, and intelligence levels for the longest time possible. Feeling a bit skeptical? Who could blame you? After years of contradictory information about the best methods for achieving brain health, it's easy to think that intermittent fasting is also just another flash-in-the-pan fad. But the big difference between intermittent fasting and other methods is evidence. There's plenty of scientific data to back up claims that intermittent fasting actually benefits the brain in a measurable, tangible way, and even more importantly, there are thousands of cases, current and historical, that show us the importance of fasting for a better, stronger, and more durable brain.

Let's take a look at just how intermittent fasting improves brain function:

Intermittent fasting works primarily by slowing the brain (and body's) aging process by bringing rampant inflammation to a screeching halt. Think about this: eating is largely a very inflammatory process. Every time you sit down and enjoy a meal, you're inadvertently setting off a series of reactions within not just your body but your mind. The most important of these reactions is that your blood sugar levels begin to rise. Now, this takes place the most when you eat high-carb or sugar-laden foods, but it is also an in-built part of the metabolic process, so even healthy foods such as legumes or certain vegetables won't protect you from a slight rise in blood glucose levels.

When blood sugar rises, it causes a whole array of unwanted and ominous side effects, but its most deadly effect is its ability to increase levels of pro-inflammatory cytokines. Pro-inflammatory cytokines act as messengers, spreading the burning fire of inflammation throughout your system, and essentially wreaking havoc on your brain's health and stability. Because pro-inflammatory cytokines literally light up your brain with inflammation, it's vital to stop them before they burn out your most important organ!

Luckily, this is easily done by practicing intermittent fasting. Research has shown that each time you fast, you effectively suppress these dangerous pro-inflammatory cytokines and put a stop to their destructive actions while at the same time promoting the production of anti-inflammatory cytokines which cool the flame and soothe the brain.

Another risk associated with the rise of blood sugar that comes from too much or improperly timed eating is a shrinking brain! Yes, that is the disturbing truth: elevated blood sugar levels can actually cause your brain's hippocampus to dry up and shrink. Considering that the hippocampus is your brain's memory center, you can see how serious the threat of a shrunken one can be!

In a groundbreaking German study, a group of more than 100 test subjects were evaluated to determine hippocampus size, as well as their blood sugar levels and ability to learn and remember. What researchers discovered was absolutely astounding: there was a very strong link between high blood glucose levels, poor memory, lowered learning abilities, and a smaller hippocampus. Results from the individuals who participated in the study displayed a clear fact: the higher a person's blood sugar levels, the smaller that person's hippocampus was likely to be, and the less able they were to learn and retain new information. The individuals who had the lowest blood sugar levels were also found to have a larger, healthier hippocampus as well as better memories and cognitive abilities!

How many times have you heard the phrase "All that sugar will rot your brain"? Well, these results prove that saying is true. Elevations in blood glucose levels associated with caloric intake are definitely connected to brain shrinkage, loss of memory, and a loss of the ability to learn new information. We now know that intermittent fasting works to significantly lower blood sugar levels and keep them within a lower range continuously. This may come as a shock to most people. Certainly, for far too long, we've been fed the myth that eating small, frequent meals several times throughout the day is the best way to control blood sugar and keep the mind in optimal health. The truth however, is very different.

Research and experience have both taught us what many people have suspected for years—high meal frequency is not the answer. If it was, the millions of people who take their doctor's advice and eat evenly spaced little meals and snacks throughout the day would not be at risk of blood sugar mediated dementia. Instead, dementia and other brain disorders are at epidemic levels, and we are only now finally beginning to see that eating fewer, less frequent meals (regardless of caloric intake) actually lowers blood sugar levels and successfully protects the brain.

It's time to start ignoring that old wives' tale advising you to eat a small meal every couple of hours. Those who have ended up on the "small, frequent meals" bandwagon are actually stoking high blood sugar levels, sparking serious inflammation, and setting up their minds for a massive meltdown. Eating too many times a day can trigger insulin resistance, glucose intolerance, and speed up the process of aging, while also bringing on dementia and cognitive disorders. This is the most destructive thing you could do to your mind and your body, and it completely goes against everything we know about the way our ancestors lived.

During the days of hunting and gathering, we weren't continually grazing on an endless supply of meals and snacks. In fact, we went through long periods of not eating, as we searched for the next meal or strived to conserve our limited supplies to eat them when we needed them most. Just because huge amounts of food are now easily available to us doesn't mean that we should be eating all day. The opposite is true—we should be mimicking the normal cycle of fasting and feeding that our brains have always experienced.

Using intermittent fasting allows you to mimic this cycle to guard yourself from terrible brain disorders and think more clearly, quickly, and effectively than ever before. It's important to note that intermittent fasting's benefits don't end at simply lowering inflammation and blood sugar levels. In fact, perhaps the most powerful ways in which it boosts brain power is through its ability to cause limited stress to the brain. Now, when I say stress, I'm not talking about the "worried, anxious, keyed up" type of stress that has been proven to be harmful to the brain. Instead, I mean the low-level, mild, and beneficial stress that fasting places on the brain cells, in the same way that working out places limited, positive stress on the muscles. Just like exercise, although it may cause momentary strain, it quickly results in improved strength and wellness.

Anytime you reduce the energy you take in for a period of time longer than 5-6 hours, you begin to positively affect the growth of brain neurons. These bouts of fasting also directly result in higher levels of

Human Growth Hormone (HGH). When men fast for 24 hours, they experience an astonishing 2000% increase in HGH levels, while women who do the same experience a 1300% increase in levels of circulating HGH!

This is important because a rush of HGH optimizes your metabolism and burns fat while simultaneously saving protein. In this way, the saved proteins get used to enhance the processing of neurons, the maintenance of collagen, the lowering of triglycerides, and the improvement of HDL cholesterol levels. All of these things contribute to a healthy mind.

We know that HGH is the exact polar opposite of the hormone insulin. While insulin is intensely pro-inflammatory, HGH is extremely anti-inflammatory. While insulin plays a role in some of the most destructive disorders mankind has developed today, HGH is a life-giving, rejuvenating, and anti-aging hormone that repairs damaged tissues, douses inflammation, and allows the brain to enter a state of "neuronal autophagy" where it cleans out any toxic debris and returns itself to the ultimate level of functioning. Because of this, when HGH is increased through even short periods of fasting, the brain-destroying processes unleashed by insulin releases are cancelled out.

Conversely, every time food is eaten, causing a release of insulin to be required, HGH production is suppressed, and all of those wonderful brain-boosting benefits it provides are eliminated. Basically, eating interrupts that extremely healthy cleansing autophagy process that HGH induces, and when it's interrupted, the brain begins to destroy itself!

So why is fasting the only way to increase and protect HGH production? Wouldn't a low-carb diet be sufficient since proteins and fats don't cause insulin spikes in the same way that carb-heavy meals do? Well, the answer to that is while proteins and fats may not spike your insulin like a bowl of pasta will, they also don't necessarily do your HGH levels any favors either. The simple truth is that eating, in and of itself, has a suppressing effect on HGH. That's why it's extremely important to give your brain "food breaks" where it can briefly enjoy the benefits of low insulin levels and increased HGH.

I know what you're thinking—HGH sounds pretty good but is it really worth skipping meals in order to increase it? To put any doubts to rest about this awesome brain-saving super hormone, let's take a quick look at the long list of amazing rewards HGH can offer your brain's functioning and health!

- HGH boosts the growth of peripheral dendrites in your brain, helping you to maintain the vital connections between your brain cells.
- It stimulates the growth of glial cells that are in charge of nourishing your brain's neurons.

- It helps your brain cells not only to repair themselves, but also to duplicate!

- It improves the myelin sheath that covers your entire central nervous system, keeping your mind safe from a myriad of deadly degenerative diseases like multiple sclerosis.

- Studies show us that when HGH levels increase, the number of dying brain cells is sharply decreased.

- We're seeing evidence that substantially increasing your HGH levels can not only prevent the development of Parkinson's, Alzheimer's, and other degenerative conditions in the first place, it can actually **REVERSE** some of their most troubling symptoms and may also slow their progression.

- HGH prevents the formation of dangerous enzymes called proteases by knocking out the free radicals that cause them.

- Research shows that HGH spurs on the release of endorphins in the brain, triggering better learning and enhancing the mood.

- Additionally, it's been shown to be at least as effective as Prozac and other anti-depressant medications in combatting depression and encouraging a lifted and more stable mood. This may be the secret behind the increase in cases of depression in older people. As we know, amounts of circulating HGH dramatically drop as we age, but intermittent fasting can get these levels back up to normal, without any harmful or costly prescription meds!

If that impressive list isn't enough to make you consider giving intermittent fasting a try, think about this: lower inflammation, stable blood sugar, and HGH production are not the only ways that fasting protects your mind and gives you a clear edge when it comes to thinking, learning, and remembering.

<u>Fasting and BDNF</u>

BDNF (Brain-Derived Neurotrophic Factor) is a critical protein that has an important effect on all of your brain's functions and also regulates your peripheral nervous system. This substance is so effective at boosting the brain that it has actually been called "miracle-grow for the mind" by Harvard psychiatrist, John J. Ratey!

It plays a vital role in everything from helping in new neuronal growth (neurogenesis), halting brain cell death, and supporting synapse growth among other functions. Because BDNF is so essential for optimal cognitive functioning, when levels of it dip, all kinds of problematic conditions arise, including premature memory loss, depression, rapid aging, psychiatric disorders like schizophrenia, and impaired neural development. Low BDNF is one of the main characteristics of Huntington's disease, and is also linked to the development of obesity, which in turn can cause a shrunken hippocampus.

BDNF works by attaching to the receptor in your brain's synapses. Once inside your brain cells, it also causes you to create even more BDNF and increases serotonin production. This particular neurotrophin may be just one among many that influence the brain, but it is also arguably the most important in preventing disease, preserving the brain, and helping it to work at the best possible levels.

Basically, a brain without sufficient amounts of BDNF is a dysfunctional mess, and making sure you have high enough amounts of it is truly one of the most beneficial moves you can make for your brain's short and long term health.

There are several ways to protect yourself from the many dangers posed by a lack of this neurotrophin, including supplements, dietary restrictions, and exercise, but the very best method of increasing BDNF is actually also one of the easiest to carry out—intermittent fasting. While restricting your calories alone can help you bolster the BDNF in your brain, nothing works quite as well as using scheduled bouts of fasting.

Every time you fast, your brain increases BDNF signaling and rolls back much of the damage that your cells and synapses have already experienced. Neurotransmission begins to function properly, disease is fought off and your entire mind begins to think work and even feel better! This method is super easy to pull off because it doesn't involve tedious "mind exercises" or regular supplementation—instead, you simply give food a miss for a short period and start reaping the rewards very quickly.

I'd like to highlight the importance of using fasting to boost your BDNF for you with a little fact: Did you know that thousands of people who have suffered traumatic events and are left suffering from Post-Traumatic Stress Disorder (PTSD) have successfully used fasting-mediated BDNF to heal their minds, moods, and lives, when medication, therapy, and other conventional methods haven't worked for them? Doctors believe this may have a lot to do with BDNF's intensively anti-inflammatory properties. In fact, BDNF is so anti-inflammatory that increased levels of it have been shown to reverse asthma, arthritis, and other inflammation-led diseases!

Intermittent Fasting and Depression:

Fasting intermittently does much more than ward off physical disorders of the brain. It also works wonders for those suffering from depression. One study found that after just a short period of fasting, 86% of depression patients experienced complete remission of their condition. Anecdotally, many of those who first try intermittent fasting are bowled over by the weight loss, decreased cravings, and mental clarity that it provides, but soon they also begin to notice an unexpected side effect—an elevated mood and a peaceful, stable, motivated state of mind. Even those who've suffered from deep anxiety for many years have reported feeling amazing benefits after only their first fast.

Now that we've looked at how intermittent fasting heals the mind, we'll be exploring one of its most famous attributes—rejuvenating you inside and out!

Chapter 9: Intermittent Fasting: Nature's Secret To Turning Back The Clock And Aging Backwards!

What if I told you that simply not eating for short periods of time, followed by eating normally, would teach your body to slow down its aging process and actually speed up its rejuvenation process? It's true!

For centuries, ancient cultures around the world have prized fasting as the secret to both lasting youth and a long, healthy life, and now science has proved them right. Both scientific research and anecdotal reports show that not only does intermittent fasting boost fat burning, banish chronic diseases, and provide better brain function, it is also the "fountain of youth" that so many of us have been dreaming of.

Research from USC has uncovered that periodically limiting food intake, even for short stretches of time, actually increases the number of progenitor and stem cells within the organs. This rejuvenating effect was seen particularly clearly in the brain, where IF caused neurons to regenerate and led to powerfully enhanced brain functions. Previous tests on mice showed that fasting intermittently promoted longevity while reducing internal and external signs of aging. In fact, in one study, mice that were made to fast intermittently before returning to a normal eating plan were able to increase their lifespan by a shocking 50%! Sounds great, but we're humans, right?

Well, fortunately, groundbreaking tests on humans have found that when we fast intermittently, even for just one or two days a week, a whole slew of exciting, life prolonging and youth promoting effects take place! One of the first things that researchers found was that IF slashed the belly fat levels of the human fasters. This is important because dangerous visceral fat often winds its way around the vital organs in the abdominal area, crushing these delicate organs and causing bruising, scarring, and eventually deadly illnesses. When this visceral fat is basically obliterated by intermittent fasting, it literally adds years to an individual's lifespan.

And the results don't end there. Intermittent fasting was also found to decrease the incidence of nearly all types of cancer, improve the immune system's functioning, and reduce inflammation, while causing them to cleanse and renew themselves through the deeply beneficial action of cell autophagy. In addition to this, common signs of aging, such as bone mineral density loss, a sluggish metabolism, and a decreased ability to remember and learn were all wiped off the map! Intermittent fasting also lowered the levels of the hormone IGF-I in the test participants. While IGF-I is essential for growth during early human development, in adulthood, it leads to higher rates of rapid aging and has even been linked to the development of cancer.

At the same time, fasting intermittently also raised levels of the anti-aging hormone IGFBP-- while reducing biomarkers such as C-reactive protein, trunk fat, and glucose, which are all linked to the development of cardiovascular disease and diabetes.

While many other weight loss and health programs can end up increasing an individual's aging process by rapidly destroying bone mass and eliminating healthy lean muscle mass along with any weight lost, intermittent fasting was shown to protect bone density while even increasing lean muscle mass, leading to an overall stronger, more balanced, younger, and fitter appearance in intermittent fasters.

Essentially, when each faster went without food, their bodies began to implement a number of genetic repair functions, switched on by the release of human growth hormone (HGH). As we know, HGH is the opposite of insulin, and while intermittent fasting decreases the highly aging hormone insulin, it boosts levels of anti-aging HGH, which leads to improved skin, lower inflammation levels, faster healing cuts, and even reduced wrinkles.

In total, it appeared that all of the human test participants in these intermittent fasting tests were not only **not actively aging,** they seemed to be **aging backwards**—regenerating and enhancing all of their bodies' cells, systems, and functions!

Intermittent Fasting Reverses Aging, Inside and Out!

Anecdotally, I've personally seen cases where many people start fasting intermittently for other health concerns, but find that their physical appearance improves so much that family and friends even think they've had cosmetic work done on their skin. They're always surprised by this side effect of IF, but I tell them that with this healing method, cell rejuvenation is happening in every cell of every organ in their bodies, including the largest of all organs, their skin! If intermittent fasting is renewing you on the inside, it only makes sense that the results would show on the outside.

One case in particular involved a man in his early 50's who had begun fasting intermittently to control his spiraling type 2 diabetes. Before fasting, he had several signs on his face of the illness that was raging within his body. These included deep lines on his forehead and around his mouth, blotchy red, angry looking skin that was prone to irritation, and in particular, large dark circles and big bags under his eyes. He had dismissed these as simply the normal signs of the aging process and hadn't believed that there was anything that could be done about them. However, it was easy to recognize that these symptoms of rapid aging were due to his uncontrolled internal illness. After all, a major part of aging is actually the wearing out of the organs and the cells that make them up through time and chronic inflammation.

The intermittent fasting worked to first douse the fire of inflammation inside him, and then to lower his insulin resistance, reversing his diabetes, and he began to see his skin improve drastically. After continuing to fast one or two days a week for several months, he became the beneficiary of constantly boosted HGH levels that smoothed his wrinkles, allowed for youthful collagen production, and calmed redness and irritation. However, those stubborn black circles and bags under his eyes remained for longer, as I knew they would. This is because they were signs of the sustained damage his kidneys had suffered during his long illness with diabetes and it would take more time to heal and rebalance these organs. After nearly a year in which he had fasted intermittently for one or two days every week, he was examined by his doctor and found that his kidney's blood urea nitrogen (BUN) levels, which had been far too high due to his diabetes, were now beginning to normalize. Slowly, the circles and bags around his eyes began to fade, and when they had completely vanished, he had his kidneys tested again. The results showed that his BUN levels were finally healthy again and that his kidneys functioned properly. Intermittent fasting had helped to heal his organs, but in doing so, it had also helped to erase and reverse the rapid aging he had been going through because of his illness! Because your body's entire system is intrinsically interwoven, fasting intermittently works in one area while also producing amazing benefits in another.

How Intermittent Fasting Kills Cancer Cells:

One of the most critical ways that intermittent fasting prolongs human life and protects the quality of that life is by killing cancer cells. Tragically, cancer has become the scourge of our times, and is now one of the leading causes of illness and death globally, particularly in older population segments. For years, doctors and researchers sought high and low for the elusive "cure for cancer" but research now shows us that it may have been right under our noses all this time. IF's ability to lay siege to and completely destroy cancer cells makes it one of the most radically effective methods of cancer therapy that we have ever seen.

Fasting intermittently works on cancer cells by literally starving them to death. But unlike chemotherapy, which also targets and kills cancer cells, IF does not harm any of the surrounding healthy cells. So just why are cancer cells especially vulnerable to fasting? Our healthy cells have the ability to switch into "survival mode" when a stressor like fasting takes place, and this mode helps them not only to make it through any fasting periods but to actually become healthier and more efficient during it.

Cancer cells are not healthy normal cells so they do not have this ability. Because they can't go into survival mode when fasting occurs, they keep on functioning in their same inefficient way and they quickly run out of the glucose they need for fuel. In this way, they are essentially starved to death by intermittent fasting!

And as if that wasn't good enough, fasting intermittently even protects and boosts the surrounding normal cells so that, if the patient does end up undergoing chemotherapy, only weakened cancer cells will be destroyed and all healthy cells will survive it intact! And there's plenty of evidence pointing to IF as the most promising natural cancer treatment yet. Let's take a look at some of these astonishing results:

One of the first studies into IF as a viable cancer treatment occurred in the 1980's. It took 48 mice and split them up into two groups of 24 mice each. One group of mice ate freely and normally for one week while the second group fasted intermittently on alternate days. Researchers then injected both groups with breast cancer. Nine days after these injections, only 5 of the mice that ate freely were still alive. When it came to the mice that had fasted intermittently however, it was a totally different story—16 out of 24 of them remained alive.

That was the first signal that IF had the power to destroy cancer cells and keep people alive. In a second study, mice with cancerous tumors were either fed normally or made to fast intermittently before receiving chemotherapy treatment. While 50 % of the mice that didn't fast died from chemotherapy toxicity, every single mouse that had been made to fast intermittently survived! Other tests show that even infrequently fasting intermittently slows down and reverses the growth of tumors. Intermittent fasting has been proved to be a powerfully targeted treatment against some of the biggest killers of the modern world, including breast cancer, prostate cancer, and even pancreatic cancer!

From ancient beliefs about fasting's power to rejuvenate the body, mind, and appearance, and prolong life, to modern-day research showing that intermittent fasting cools inflammation, eliminates visceral fat, banishes deadly diseases, and even causes the cells to renew themselves, the evidence just can't be ignored. Intermittent fasting is the highly effective secret to achieving a long, healthy and youthful life!

Chapter 10:The Intermittent Fasting and Exercise Connection: Double Your Weight Loss, Enhance Anti-Aging, Fight Disease, and Sharpen Your Mind With These Simple Tips!

While intermittent fasting is incredibly powerful on its own, combining it with the appropriate exercise routine can amplify every single one of its benefits. If you're looking for intense effects that you can't get with any other method, read on for the secret to rapid weight loss and magnified anti-aging, anti-inflammatory, and pro-health, and longevity results!

The "Eat Before You Exercise" Myth

We're often told that it's important to eat before exercising, to provide stable energy during the workout period and to help keep dizziness and exhaustion at bay. We're even told that exercising on empty is one of the most detrimental actions you can take against your body. The truth is the absolute opposite. The fact is that eating shortly before working out can actually harm you by causing an intense spike in your blood sugar levels, which will then be followed by a severe plunge. On the other hand, there's really no limit to the amazing benefits you can gain from working out while in the midst of a fast.

Maximize Your Fat Burning Workout

If you're like most people, you want to get the very most out of the time and effort that you put into exercising, and if that's the case, then working out while in a fasting state is certainly the best way to achieve the highest payoff possible. Any time you hit the gym or track while intermittently fasting, your body is literally forced into losing fat mass. This is because your body's ability to lose weight is under the control of your sympathetic nervous system (SNS). This system is, in turn, switched on whenever you exercise on an empty stomach.

In addition, the super-combination of fasting and working out actually intensifies the effects of cellular catalysts and factors that force your body to begin breaking down glycogen stores and fat stores in order to gain energy. Research has found that when you fast before you perform aerobic exercise, you actually lose more weight, and specifically, more body fat than you would if you exercised in a non-fasting state.

Rejuvenate Yourself Even Faster, By Exercising While Fasting

We already know that intermittent fasting is a veritable fountain of youth, but if you thought that its wonderful benefits couldn't possibly be improved upon, you were wrong. If you work out while fasting, it produces a state known as acute oxidative stress, and this kind of positive stress leads to an increased development of muscle mass. Fasting and exercise achieve this by stimulating your mitochondria to produce beneficial substances such as superoxide dismutase and glutathione. It also causes your muscles to be able to withstand exhaustion and to use energy more efficiently and effectively. So, in effect, when you work out while fasting, far from harming your muscle mass, you actually revitalize your muscles and cause them to become "younger" in both form and function.

Renew Your Brain With Intermittent fasting and Exercise

When taken together, exercise and intermittent fasting make up the most potent form of therapy for your mind. Each time you exercise without eating, you turn on muscle regulatory factors (MRFs) and brain-derived neurotrophic factor (BDNF). These growth factors and genes tell your brain stem cells to turn into brand new neurons. In this way, every workout you engage in during your intermittent fasting period is actually "turning back time" on your brain, renewing it and making it youthful again.

High Intensity Interval Training: Give Your Intermittent Fast Routine A Real "HIIT" of Power

If you're aiming to get rid of a large amount of weight in a short amount of time and you want to achieve an excellent muscle-to-fat ratio, pairing intermittent fasting with high intensity interval training (also known as HIIT) is definitely the best bet!

Some of the numerous rewards you can expect to reap include:

- Super-efficient fat burning mechanisms
- Rapid and lasting weight loss
- A higher ratio of muscle to fat
- Improved body shape
- Higher levels of human growth hormone (HGH)
- Improved cognitive abilities and a younger brain
- Improved or reversed depression

In addition:

- HIIT exercises actually help you burn up to an additional 15 % more calories than you would if you were doing normal exercises! Who wouldn't want that?
- With HIIT, you continue to burn a large amount of calories even after your workout is done.
- HIIT workouts actually provide better outcomes in preventing and reversing cardiovascular conditions than normal workouts. Research shows that HIIT can help keep hearts in shape more effectively and for longer than other exercise types.
- HIIT has been found to offer you higher levels of energy and optimized fat burning.

If this sounds like something you definitely want to try, you need no fancy equipment or special training. In fact, HIIT is a pretty simple concept to take in. All you have to do is first warm-up and then follow this with an intense burst of cardio activity that lasts for

30 seconds. You then follow this with a full recovery period of 90 seconds. The most important thing to remember is to breathe properly while working out and also to give it your maximum effort when it comes to the 30 second bursts of cardio. This can be done for up to 20 minutes a day with any kind of cardio-based activity, including running or on a stationary bike.

Which Types Of Intermittent Fasting Go Best With HIIT?

I recommend trying to combine HIIT with all methods of intermittent fasting, if you're healthy and fit enough to do so. It goes exceptionally well with any type of IF, from 5:2 to the Warrior fast, and any modified versions of these fasts. However, with Eat Stop Eat fasting, it's recommended that you engage in weight training rather than HIIT or any other type of cardio.

The Warrior Fast and Exercise

Exercise plays a role in the Warrior fast method so it was important to include a brief note on it. When on this fasting method, you are advised to work out during the under-eating or fasting stage of your day. All exercise on the Warrior fast should be brief and very intense, totaling no more than about half an hour. Exercises that work out your entire body such as sprints, squats, kicks, jumps, and chin-ups are favored over any type of targeted exercise moves.

CFT: Work Out Until You Can't Work Out Any More On the Warrior Fast

With the Warrior fast, the idea of CFT, or controlled fatigue training, is crucial. With this method, you are encouraged to work out when fatigue has already begun to set in, allowing your body to spark the survival reaction through your sympathetic nervous system. This effectively copies the way ancient warriors would have kept up physical movement during battle, even when totally worn out and ready to drop. Pushing yourself to the limit a few times a week provides an enhanced positive stress response that really draws out every last benefit of the Warrior fast.

The Exception to The Rule: Why It's Important To Eat Right After A Heavy Lifting Exercise Routine

It's vital that you eat within half an hour of doing heavy lifting exercises because doing so aids in muscle building and also provides support to weary muscles, allowing them to recover from your workout session. It's important to make sure that your post-heavy lifting meal encompasses a source of fast-assimilating protein, such as whey with water, yogurt, or kefir.

As you begin to work out in a fasted state more and more, you will notice that your ability to withstand it increases exponentially and that you can actually feel the enhanced fat burning taking place!

Conclusion: The Takeaway

First of all, allow me to thank you for taking this journey of knowledge with me and reaching the end of this book! Congratulations on saying NO to ill health, NO to stubborn weight gain, depression, dementia, and premature aging, and a resounding NO to the idea that we can't heal our bodies and minds naturally!

When I first sat down to write this guide to understanding and using the secrets of intermittent fasting, it was with individuals like yourself in mind— those who are not satisfied with the status quo, with doing what they have always been told to, and who are not willing to give up on their desire for intense health, vitality, fitness, mental clarity, and longevity, just because conventional medicine and nutrition tell them it's impossible. If you've already begun fasting intermittently, you've no doubt begun to *see* and *feel* the amazing effects that I talk about in this book. As you continue on your path to achieving lifelong vigor and wellness, remember that you are travelling down an ancient, tried, and true way of wellness.

I urge you to use this guide as a point of reference. When people question you about using intermittent fasting, you'll be able not only to point to the visible changes in your body, appearance, and energy levels, but will have all of the scientific evidence on hand to show that this ancient way of eating, living, and healing works just as well today as it did centuries ago!

In closing, I'd like to wish you the very best on your road to repairing, rejuvenating, and protecting every cell in your body and mind, and would like to remind you to check out the recipe index at the end of this book for a selection of delicious, truly nourishing meal options to use with the different types of intermittent fasting we explored in this guide!

Good luck and great health!

****

****

Recipe Index

Meal Options for 5:2 Fast

Total calorie allowance for fast days: Approximately 500-600

Fast Day Meal Options (Combine any 2 options you'd like, as long as they total no more than 500-600 calories.)

1. Mid-day snack option: 1 apple, sliced, with 1 tablespoon of almond butter and a pinch of ground cinnamon. (142 calories)

2. Mid-day snack option: Handful of plums in plain Greek yogurt. (140 calories)

3. Mid-day snack option: Half a cup of raspberries and 100 grams of plain Greek yogurt. (92 calories)

4. Evening meal option: Miso soup. (30 calories)

5. Mid-day or evening meal option: 2 soft boiled eggs on a bed of baby spinach leaves and 25 grams of feta sprinkled over and lemon to taste. (252 calories)

6. Mid-day or evening meal option: 100 grams of turkey or ham over 4 sticks of asparagus and 1 tablespoon of balsamic vinegar. (158 calories)

7. Mid-day or evening meal option: 200 grams of smoked salmon and 1 cup of spinach, cooked and seasoned with salt and a squeeze of lemon. (275 calories)

8. Mid-day or evening meal option: 3 scrambled eggs with 1 tablespoon of olive oil. (320 calories)

9. Mid-day snack option: 1 cup of plain, traditional kefir. (135 calories)

10. Mid-day snack option: Fresh Green Juice: 4 celery sticks, 1 apple, 1 cucumber, 6 pieces of kales and a squeeze of lime. (205 calories)

11. Mid-day or evening meal option: 200 grams minced turkey sautéed with half a red onion, garlic, and black pepper. (289 calories)

12. Mid-day or evening meal option: Sautee together 40 grams of beets, 6 pieces of asparagus, and 130 grams of turkey breast steak, seasoned with salt and black pepper. (220 calories)

13. Place in oven and roast together 1 zucchini, 1 cup of mushrooms, ½ of medium bell pepper, and 1 red onion. Add 1 tablespoon balsamic vinegar and 1 tablespoon grass-fed butter and season with salt and black pepper. (301 calories)

14. Mid-day or evening meal option: 1 chicken breast grilled in 2 teaspoon of honey, salt and black pepper, grated ginger, and squeeze of lemon. (202 calories)

15. Mid-day snack option: ½ cup of blueberries. (41 calories)

****
****

16. Fasting Coffee Recipe (As Promised, Enjoy!!)

To make a delicious cup of IF fat burning, metabolism boosting, concentration enhancing, energy-giving coffee…..

- 1 cup of fresh high quality coffee
- 1 tablespoon of grass-fed butter
- 1 tablespoon of pure coconut oil
- A pinch of salt
- A pinch of ground cinnamon, to taste

Instructions: Blend all ingredients together on high speed until the mixture is frothy. Drink immediately and enjoy!

Recipes:

These low carb meals can be used for the Warrior fast, the 24 Hour fast, and the 16/8 fast. Don't worry about portions of calories, as these fasting methods do not require you to do so.

Note: If you are using the Warrior fast method, each meal can be adapted by choosing the leanest cuts of meat or switching to chicken breast where desired. Some recipes may contain combinations not recommended on the Warrior fast, and have been marked "not for Warrior fast" in such cases.

17. Warrior Fast Green Salad:

(Can be eaten with all fasting methods)

- 6 bunches of kale
- 1 handful of baby spinach
- 1 handful of shredded basil
- 1 yellow onion, diced

- 2 handfuls of cherry tomatoes
- ¼ cup of fresh mushrooms

Olive oil vinaigrette

- ½ of a lemon
- 9 tablespoons of pure olive oil
- 4 tablespoons of pure balsamic vinegar
- Salt and pepper to taste

Instructions: Add all salad ingredients to large salad bowl. In a separate container, whisk olive oil, balsamic vinegar, salt and pepper, and squeeze of lemon together. Pour vinaigrette over salad and mix all ingredients thoroughly.

18. Mediterranean Baked Eggs

- 6 eggs
- Handful of chopped basil
- 1 teaspoon of dried oregano
- 4 tablespoons of grass-fed butter
- 1 medium yellow onion, roughly chopped
- 2 handfuls of olives
- ½ a red bell pepper chopped up
- 125 grams of crumbled feta cheese
- Salt and pepper to taste

Instructions: Whisk eggs together with oregano, salt and pepper in bowl. In a pan, sauté the onions in butter until golden, then toss in the bell pepper, basil, and onions.

Pour the egg mixture into the pan and allow to cook until slightly runny. Crumble the feta cheese over the eggs and place into the stove to cook until firm for about 5 minutes.

19. Sizzling Chicken Breast, Mushroom and Bell Pepper Stir-Fry

- 3 large chicken breasts, grilled and sliced into strips
- 2 small red onions, finely chopped
- 9 tablespoons olive oil
- ½ cup cooked spinach
- ½ cup of fresh shitake mushrooms
- 1 large green bell pepper cut into long strips
- 1 teaspoon finely minced garlic
- 1 teaspoon finely minced ginger
- ½ teaspoon grated lemon peel
- ½ teaspoon cumin
- Salt and pepper to taste

- Squeeze of lemon

Instructions: In a sizzling wok, fry onions, bell peppers, and mushrooms in olive oil. Add chicken strips, cumin, garlic, ginger, lemon peel, salt, and pepper to the pan and cook at high heat. Remove from heat and serve beside spinach, adding a squeeze of lemon.

20. Loaded Avocado Cups

- 2 large avocadoes
- 1 large lemon
- 400 grams of minced beef
- Handful of chopped parsley
- 2 tablespoons olive oil
- ½ small yellow onion, diced
- ½ teaspoon minced garlic
- 2 tomatoes finely chopped
- 1 large pepper, chopped
- Salt and pepper to taste

Instructions: Peel avocadoes and slice them in half. Squeeze lemon juice over them, sprinkle with salt, and set aside.

In a pan, brown the minced beef with the onion in olive oil. Add garlic and chopped pepper, parsley and season to taste. Take off the heat and add the diced tomatoes before spooning the mixture into the halved avocado cups and serve.

21. Ginger Glazed Salmon

- 1 salmon fillet
- 1 small yellow onion, chopped
- 2 tablespoons honey
- 4 tablespoons grass-fed butter
- 1 teaspoon minced garlic
- 1 teaspoon minced ginger
- 1 teaspoon dill
- Juice of 2 small limes
- Salt and pepper, to taste

Instructions: Massage the salmon fillet with half of the butter, season it with salt, pepper, and dill. Place it on a bed of chopped onions and cook in the oven until just pink and tender in the center.

In a separate sauce pan combine the honey, juice of 2 limes, minced ginger, and minced garlic together with the butter to make a warm glaze.

Pour this glaze over the salmon and place back in the switched off oven for 3-5 minutes. Remove and serve with a simple green salad.

22. Honey Dijon & Balsamic Smoked Trout Salad

- 400 grams of smoked trout
- Warrior fast green salad (recipe above)
- 1 lemon, quartered

Dressing:

- 4 tablespoons pure Dijon mustard
- 2 tablespoons olive oil
- 2 tablespoons balsamic vinegar
- 2 tablespoons honey
- Juice from ½ small orange
- ½ teaspoon minced garlic
- ½ small red shallot finely chopped
- Pinch of salt
- Pinch of turmeric
- Pinch of black pepper

Instructions: Arrange the smoked trout on a bed of the green salad. In a separate container, whisk together the Dijon mustard, olive oil, balsamic vinegar, honey, orange juice, garlic, red shallot, and all seasoning, until the dressing is thick but still pourable. Pour this over the smoked trout and salad and serve with the quartered lemon.

23. Sweet and Satisfying Yogurt, Fruit and Nut Parfait

<u>Note: Not for Warrior fast</u>

- 1 green apple, sliced
- Handful of blueberries,
- Handful of raspberries
- Handful of blackberries
- Handful of almonds
- 300 grams of pure grass-fed yogurt
- 2 pinches of pure vanilla
- 2 pinches of ground cinnamon

Instructions: In a tall glass, alternately layer the fruit, nuts and yogurt. Sprinkle the vanilla and cinnamon on top and serve with a long spoon.

Quick Triple Berry Yogurt Smoothie

<u>Note: Not for Warrior fast</u>

- Handful of raspberries,
- Handful of blueberries
- Handful of strawberries

- 1 cup grass-fed raw yogurt
- 1 pinch of pure vanilla
- 1 pinch of salt

Instructions: Combine all ingredients in a blender or food processor and blend until thick and frothy. Serve cold or room temperature.

Stir-Fried Pepper Steak with Green Vegetables

- 1 pound beef sirloin, cut into thin strips
- 5 tablespoons olive oil
- ½ cup of broccoli
- ½ cup of cauliflower
- 3 spring onions, chopped diagonally
- 1 green bell pepper cut into thin strips
- 2 carrots cut into thin strips
- 1 ½ teaspoons grated ginger
- 1 teaspoon minced garlic
- ½ teaspoon chili powder
- 1 teaspoon toasted sesame seeds
- Salt and black pepper to season

Instructions: In a large wok, heat up the olive oil. Add beef and stir until browned, before adding in the spring onions, broccoli, cauliflower, bell pepper, carrots, ginger, and garlic and cook.

Add sesame seeds and chili powder and combine before switching off the heat. Serve hot.

Bon Appetit!

****
****

End